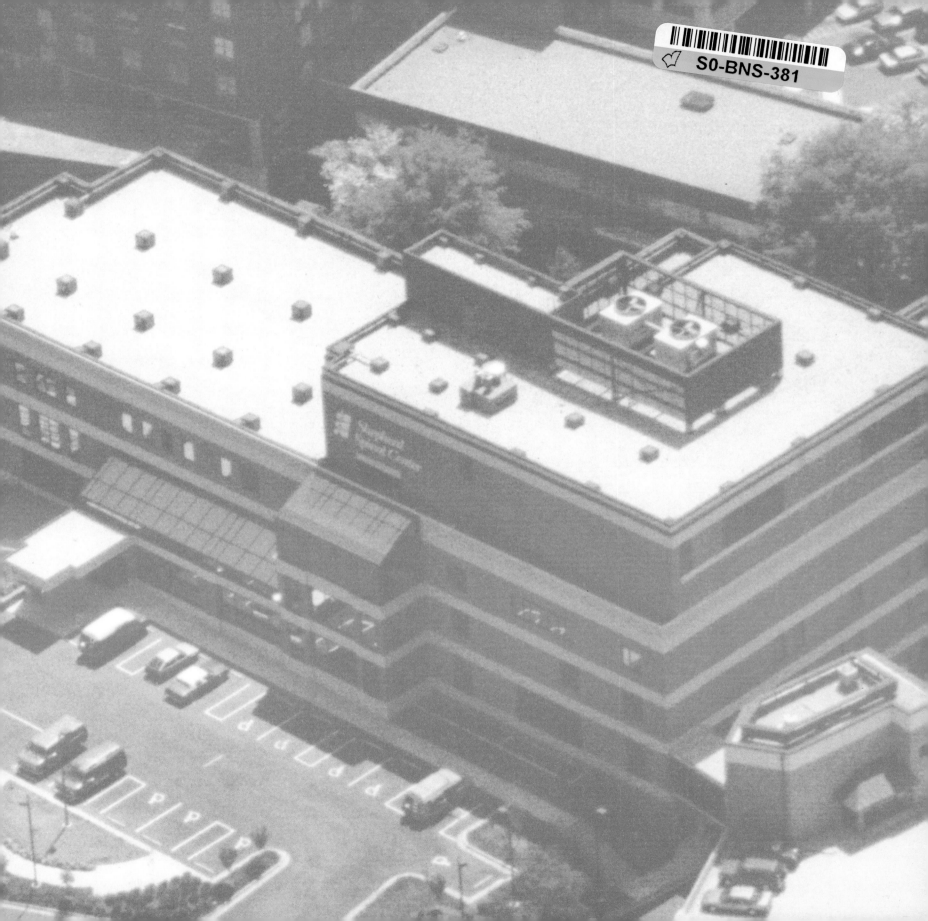

Restoring Hope
Rebuilding Lives

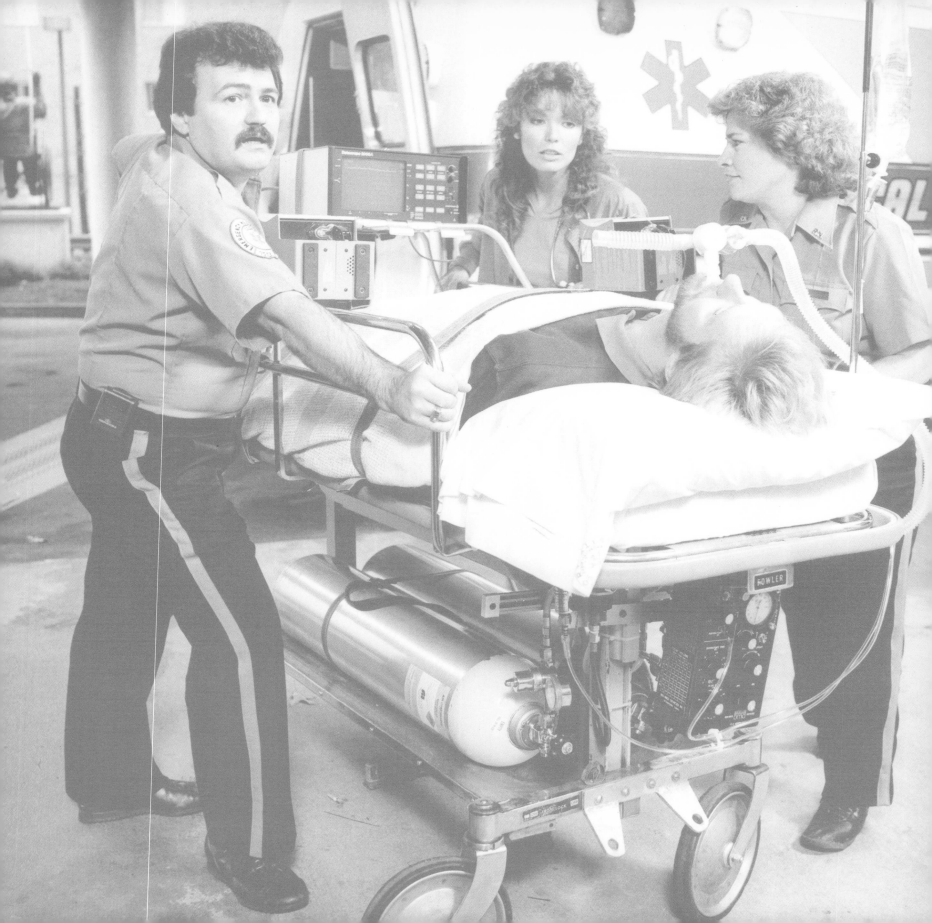

Restoring Hope
Rebuilding Lives

The Story of Shepherd Center

SHEPHERD CENTER
A Catastrophic
Care Hospital

By John Yow

Published by
Shepherd Center, Inc.
2020 Peachtree Road, NW
Atlanta, GA 30309

Printed in Korea

ISBN 0-9716494-0-5

Library of Congress
Catalog Number 2001 135945

Photography credits for following pages:
Nick Arroyo: 69
George A. Clark: ii, iv, 2, 3, 11, 15, 21, 26, 29, 30, 34-35, 40, 41, 45, 51, 53, 55, 59, 63, 68, 71, 73, 75, 78-79, 84, 91, 95, 100, 109, 110
Gittings: 129
Enid Grigg: 23, 131 (inset)
Chris Hamilton ©1996: 87
Dean Hesse: 80, 81, 83, 115, 123, 124, 127, 128, 131
Billy Howard: 18, 32, 48, 56, 60, 92, 102, 112, 118, 134
Teryl Jackson: front endsheets, 105, 121
Kathryn Kolb: 125
E. Alan McGee: back endsheets
Holly Sasnett: vi, 1, 142, 143, 144
Alana Shepherd: 16, 27
Lynne Siler: 88, 94, 97
Marilyn Suriani: 4, 9

Readers, please note: every effort was made to accurately credit all photographers for the photographs that appear within this book. Should you notice an error or omission, please contact Shepherd Center so that we may update our files.

Picture research: Monika Nikore, Julie Frazier

Designed and produced by:
Shock Design, Inc., Atlanta, Georgia
shockdesign@mindspring.com

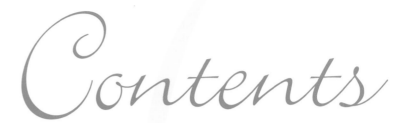

Contents

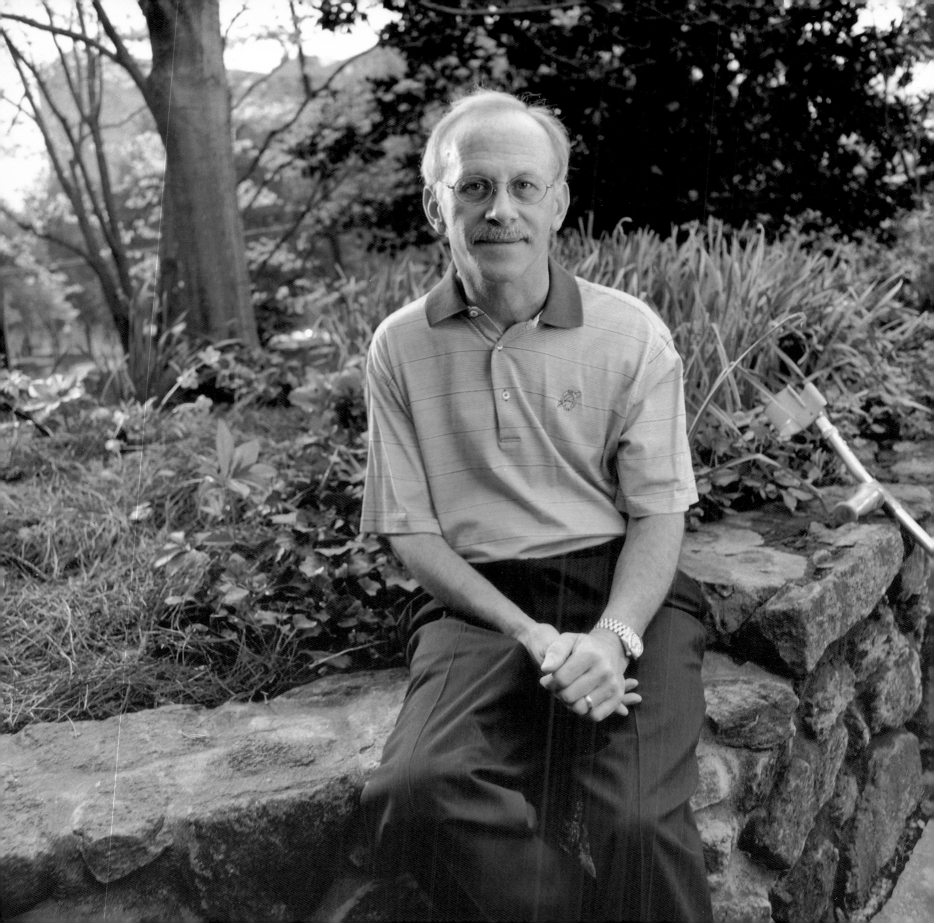

Foreword

For the success of Shepherd Center over these 25 years I have more people to thank than I could possibly name. But for the fact that I survived five weeks in Brazil, and lived to celebrate our 25th anniversary, I have a shorter list of people to thank, and I would like to share their names.

I'm alive today because of three men in Brazil: Dr. Roberto Bibas, Dr. Aloysio DeSalles Fonseca, and Adolfo Gentil. Had it not been for these three gentlemen, Shepherd Center would not be here.

Dr. Bibas, a young, brilliant thoracic surgeon of Egyptian-Jewish-Brazilian heritage, will remain indelibly etched in my mind. When most people in my condition would have been considered hopeless, he went to every extreme to keep me alive.

Likewise Dr. Aloysio DeSalles Fonseca, perhaps the best internist in Brazil, whose skills were certainly tested during my five weeks in that hospital in Rio de Janeiro.

Their job was not easy. Their nurses were overworked and exhausted; their equipment and facilities were not the best. My bed was too short, so that my feet stuck through the bed rails and had to be supported with towels to prevent "foot drop." They had to prop the head of the bed up with bricks in order to hang enough weight to get my neck straightened out to reduce the stress of the fracture. The air conditioner in my room had to run full blast to keep my fever down, which made the unit ice up. Dad and the hospital maintenance man kept having to go outside trying to thaw the coils to keep the unit running.

But it was Adolfo Gentil who worked behind the scenes to make sure our crisis did not deteriorate beyond the point of medical help. When my uncle Clyde Shepherd had overseen a Shepherd Construction Company project in Brazil some years earlier, he and Adolfo had become close friends, and it was to Adolfo that my family now turned.

During the initial stages of my hospital stay, Dad was having to get money wired down almost every other day, having to go to the bank, having to pay cash for this hospital service and that hospital service. A tremendous hassle at a time when there was already plenty of stress. But Adolfo, as soon as he got word of our trouble, came in and took charge. Not only did he make sure we had the best doctors, but he told the hospital, "Quit worrying about the money. If the bills ever get to a million dollars, call me and I'll worry about it." He gave us carte blanche to get the care I needed.

Adolfo also helped Dad get in touch with Colonel Bill Renny at the American Embassy, who secured clearance for the U.S. Air Force plane to come in and land, the plane that would finally fly me home. As soon as the plane landed, though, the radar went out, and we were told that it would be two or three weeks before technicians would be available to fix the problem. In two or three weeks, I would be dead. But Adolfo called his former secretary, who had gone to work for the president of PanAm Airlines in South America, and she arranged for their maintenance crews to take over. The plane was fixed that same day. The point is, Adolfo was the best friend we could have had, and he simply would not let us down. I am proud to say that he is my son Jamie's godfather.

While I am at it, I should also express my gratitude for Herman Talmadge's help in persuading the Air Force to requisition the Marietta-manufactured Lockheed C-141 Medivac plane. The Air Force will come to you, for free, anywhere in the world, but on their time schedule; that is, when they've got a plane coming through. Otherwise, you've got to cut through the red tape; somebody's got to walk it through and get it done. Herman Talmadge, who had been a friend of my grandfather's way back when, saw to it.

Finally, there was the flight surgeon, a woman who was smart enough and decisive enough to insist that we fly at sea level all the way home, even though it necessitated a refueling stop at "Roosevelt Roads" in Puerto Rico. This was an almost unheard-of precaution, but one that would have probably saved my life if we had for some reason lost cabin pressure during the flight.

And then I was home, very thankful to be alive, and about to embark on a new and unforeseen chapter in my life—one for which, as I say, I have many other people to thank.

I do thank all of you, who have been a part of Shepherd Center, from the bottom of my heart. I believe the blessing that came out of my five weeks in Brazil is that Shepherd Center has been able to help so many critically injured people have a recovery experience very different, and much better, than mine.

James Shepherd

Board of Directors

X

Georgia Members

Mr. Fred Aftergut
Mr. Fred V. Alias
Mrs. Carleton F. Allen
Mr. John G. Alston
Mrs. Tazwell L. Anderson, Jr.
Mr. Marvin S. Arrington
Ms. Amanda Brown-Olmstead
Ms. Marnite Calder
Mr. Michael C. Carlos
Mr. Joseph W. Chapman, Jr.
Mr. Neil J. Conrad
Mr. Dennis E. Cooper
Mr. Malon W. Courts
Mrs. John M. DeBorde III
Mrs. Samuel DuBose
Mrs. Martha M. Dykes
Mr. David O. Ellis
Mr. William B. Erb
Mrs. J.B. Fuqua
Mr. J.B. Fuqua
Mr. Thomas C. Gallagher
Mrs. Robert J. Gibson
Ms. Nancy Green
Mr. Joseph W. Hamilton, Jr.
Mrs. T. Rudy Harrell
Mr. William C. Hatcher
Mr. Robert H. Hogg III
Mr. Lindsey Hopkins III
Mr. Jerry M. Hux
Mrs. M. Douglas Ivester
Mr. Harrison Jones II
Mrs. Richard Jones
Mr. Thomas H. Kirbo
Mrs. Carl Knobloch, Jr.
Therus C. Kolff, MD
Mrs. Thomas H. Lanier
Mrs. Bernard Marcus
Mrs. Thomas O. Marshall
Mr. Philip W. Millians
Mrs. James Miller

Mrs. John O. Mitchell
Mr. Joseph Moderow
Mr. Michael Morris
Mr. Solon Patterson
Mrs. Charles Peterson
Mr. G. Joseph Prendergast
Mr. James Madison Reynolds III
Mrs. Roy Richards
Mr. James C. Richards
Mr. Lee W. Richards
Mrs. William M.Scaljon
Mr. S. Stephen Selig III
Mr. Clyde Shepherd III
Mr. Thomas C. Shepherd
Judge Marvin Shoob
Mr. John E Singleton
Mr. Steve R. Slade
Mrs. Becky Robinson Smith
Mrs. J. Lucian Smith
Mr. Spencer W. Smith, Jr.
Mrs. Jody Sodel
Mr. D. Gary Thompson
Ms. Sally G. Tomlinson
Mrs. Sharon S. Umphenour
Mrs. Mickey McQueen Webb
Mrs. John H. Weitnauer, Jr.
Mr. Mark Wietecha
Mr. Clay Willcoxon
Mrs. Thomas R. Williams
Mr. Erwin Zaban

National Members

Judge Charles Lee Allen
Judge Jennifer B. Coffman
The Honorable Bob Dole
Mr. Allen H. Higginbotham, Jr.
Mr. Travis Roy
Ms. Margaret A. Staton
Judge Charles D. Susano, Jr.
Mrs. Arnold Wright, Jr.

ACTIVE MEDICAL STAFF

David F. Apple, MD
Stephen Barnett, MD
James K. Bennett, MD
Gerald Bilsky, MD
Brock Bowman, MD
Dennis Choat, MD
Christopher Clare, MD
David DeRuyter, MD
Keith M. Dockery, MD
Jenelle E. Foote, MD
Bruce G. Green, MD
Gary Gropper, MD
Fayyaz Haq, MD
Wylly Killorin, MD
S. Robert Lathan, MD
Donald P. Leslie, MD
Allen P. McDonald, MD
Robert A. Miller, MD
John David Mullins, MD
H. Herndon Murray, MD
Allan E. Peljovich, MD
Robert W. Powers, MD
David Ripley, MD
Randy F. Rizor, MD
Kevin Rozas, MD
James A. Settle, MD
Arthur J. Simon, MD
Darrell N. Simone, MD
Douglas S. Stuart, MD
Ben W. Thrower, MD
David Walega, MD
Andrew D. Zadoff, MD

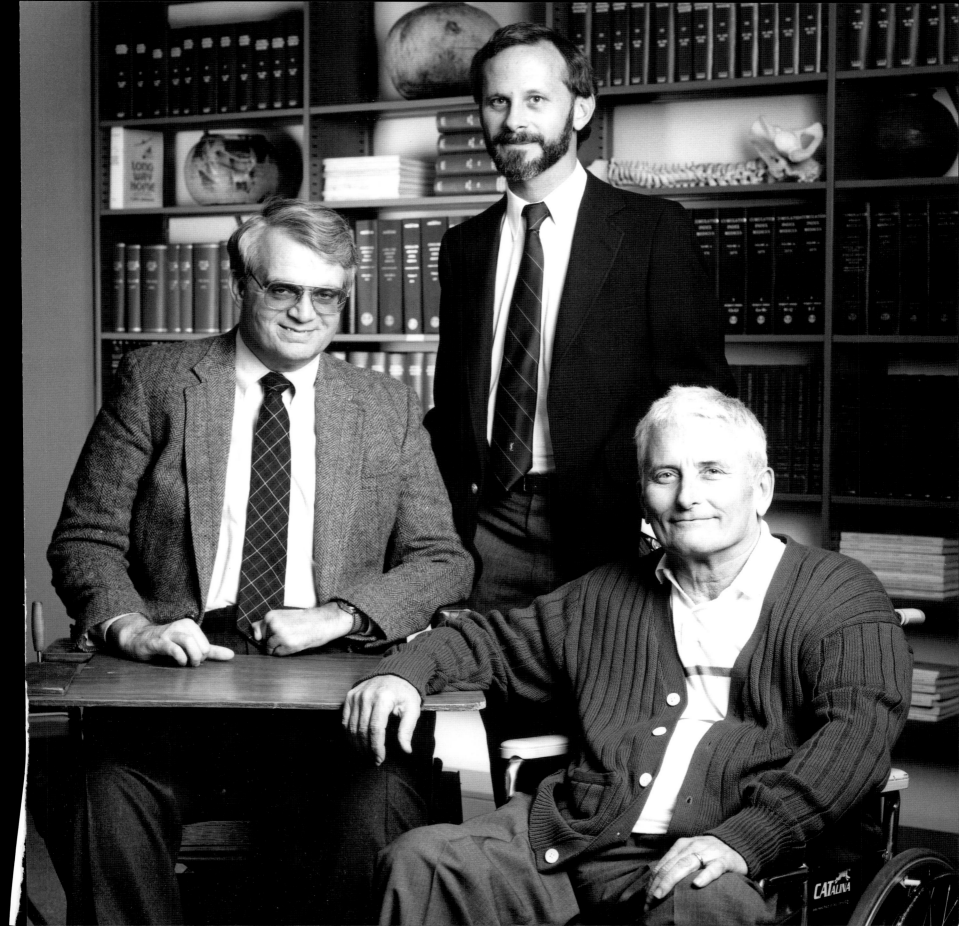

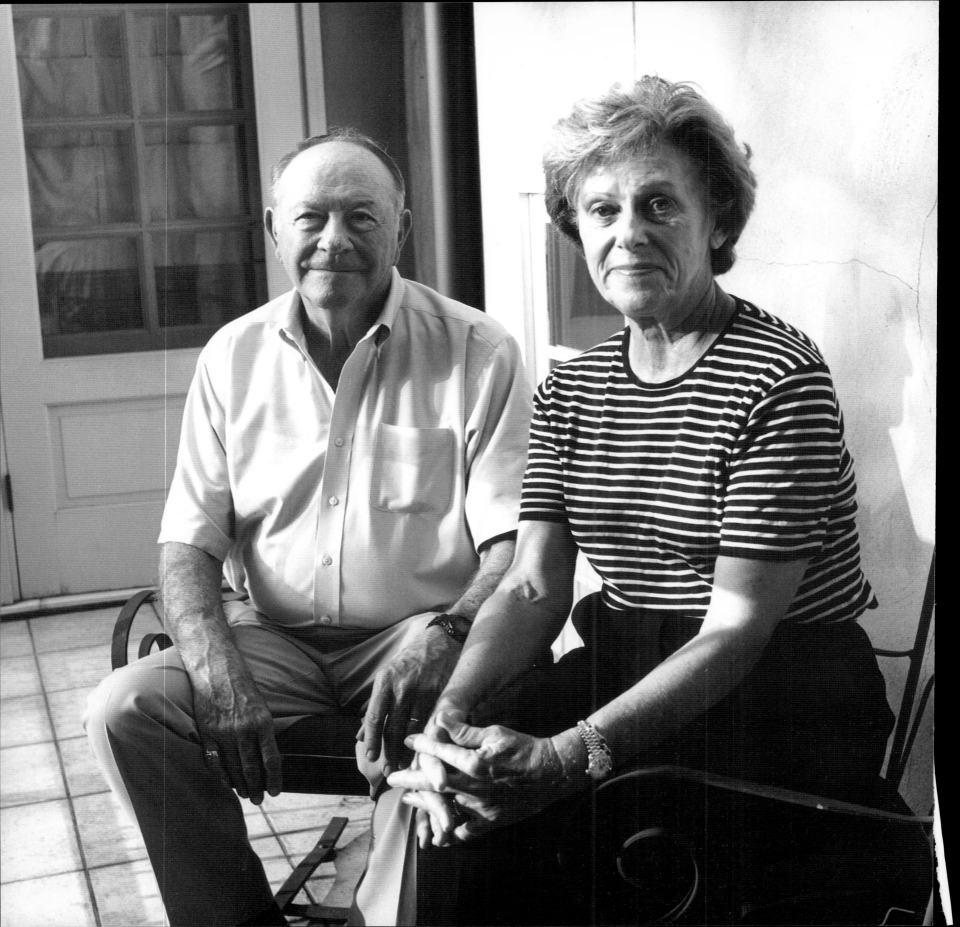

James's parents, Alana and Harold Shepherd, embraced the idea enthusiastically. After all, they had seen first-hand what Craig had done for James and had also noticed, according to Harold, that as many as a third of Craig's patients were from the Southeast. The Shepherds began recruiting, turning first to old friends in the community: Henry Smith, an architect and lifelong friend of Harold who just happened to knock on the Shepherds' door the very day they got the terrible call from Brazil; Atlanta developer and family friend Frank Carter; Virginia Crawford, the across-the-street neighbor whom Harold calls, "as good a friend as I ever had." The team was forming.

To Alana, characteristically, it was a matter of inexorable logic from "there ought to be something here" to "why not do something about it?" But James recalls one of the reasons "why not": money. Clearly, fundraising would be job one, and family and friends began contacting every individual, corporation, and foundation who might have an interest. "Mother and I talked to every garden club in Georgia for any contribution we could get," as James puts it, "and we were extremely grateful for those earliest donations." The hard work sometimes paid off unexpectedly. Henry Smith remembers approaching Ed Smith of (then) First National Bank of Atlanta: " 'Oh, I can't help you,' Ed said, but a couple of months later we got a grant from one of the foundations the bank's trust department controlled." And in some cases the work wasn't all that hard. One of Harold's favorite recollections is the call he placed to his Athens friend, Dick Budd.

" 'How much do you want me to give you?' Dick asked. I told him I couldn't tell him how much to give. Dick said, 'Okay, then, I'm gonna start counting, and you just tell me when to stop.' He started at five thousand . . . six . . . seven . . . I made him stop at ten."

To further educate the donor community, a program was conducted in the gymnasium of Atlanta's Lovett School, at which James and Clark Harrison offered themselves as examples of spinal cord injury and the possibilities of rehabilitation. Henry Smith remembers how Clark would pretend to accidentally fall out of his wheelchair and then, while everybody was going "Oh my," he would simply pull himself back into it again. "This was his way of showing people that being in a wheelchair doesn't mean you're helpless."

The dream began to take tangible shape with the hiring of Dr. David F. Apple, Jr. as medical director. One of Dr. Apple's partners, Dr. John Roberts, had been one of James's physicians during his stay at Piedmont Hospital prior to going to Denver, and Dr. Apple had gotten to know James, as he remembers, "when it was my turn to cover." Dr. Apple also credits Dr. Roberts for recommending him when the Shepherds began looking for a medical director for their dreamed-of

The Earliest Disciples

Without the dedicated and determined effort—along with the unwavering faith—of a small circle of early believers, the dream could never have come to fruition. That core group, by and large, evolved into Shepherd Center's original board of directors:

James H. Shepherd, Jr., Chairman
Virginia C. Crawford, Vice President
Ted Forbes, Jr., Corporate Secretary
Alana Shepherd, Recording Secretary
Fred Aftergut, Treasurer
John Aderhold
James Brandhorst
Conway Broun
Frank Carter
Roy Day, Jr.
Anne DeBorde
Paul Duke
Clark Harrison
J. Harold Shepherd
Henry Smith
Barrie Thrasher, MD
David Webb

5

spinal cord treatment facility. "I had had a fellowship in rehabilitation—though mainly in arthritis—as part of my training, and I was also at that time director of the Easter Seals Outpatient Center and thinking about doing something with an inpatient clinic, so the Shepherd's idea sounded very interesting to me." Not that it could have been an easy decision for a young orthopedist whose wife was about to deliver their fourth child. He was being asked to buy into nothing more tangible than a vision. According to Harold, Dr. James Funk, the head of Peachtree Orthopedic Clinic, told Dave he was crazy, that the idea would never fly. (Dr. Funk has since apologized to him, Harold adds, "but I tell him, Jimmy, don't apologize, if you told me you were going into the road building business, I'd look at you real funny, too.")

But Dr. Apple certainly looked like the right choice to James and Alana, as they sat around the table in the Shepherds' dining room —"the board room in the early days"—conducting interviews. "He took a huge gamble coming with us," James concedes, "but we gave him an opportunity to follow his real interest in rehab, which he would have had a hard time pursuing in his normal practice. I don't think he regrets it." Once on board, Dr. Apple—along with architect Henry Smith—visited rehabilitation centers throughout the country, including Craig Hospital, the one the Shepherds hoped to replicate as closely as possible.

Next to be decided was the matter of a location—no easy problem. "Just about everybody we talked to," recalls James, "gave us a flat no. They just didn't think such a facility was needed, didn't see it as a priority." But Dr. Apple knew of an empty wing in a northwest Atlanta hospital and thought its management might be interested in tenants. "They didn't understand rehab," says Dr. Apple, "but they understood empty space, so we were able to work out a deal."

So, with a medical director and one additional physician (Dr. Herndon Murray, a young Atlanta-born orthopedist with an interest in spine trauma whom Dr. Apple lured on board), with three therapists, with enough space to accommodate six patients, with nursing help from the leasing hospital, and with cheers of wild enthusiasm from the Shepherd family and friends, Shepherd Spinal Center (SSC) opened its doors on August 18, 1975—just one short year after the idea was first conceived.

And Van Knighton, still the victim of a terrible accident, was also the beneficiary of a dream made real.

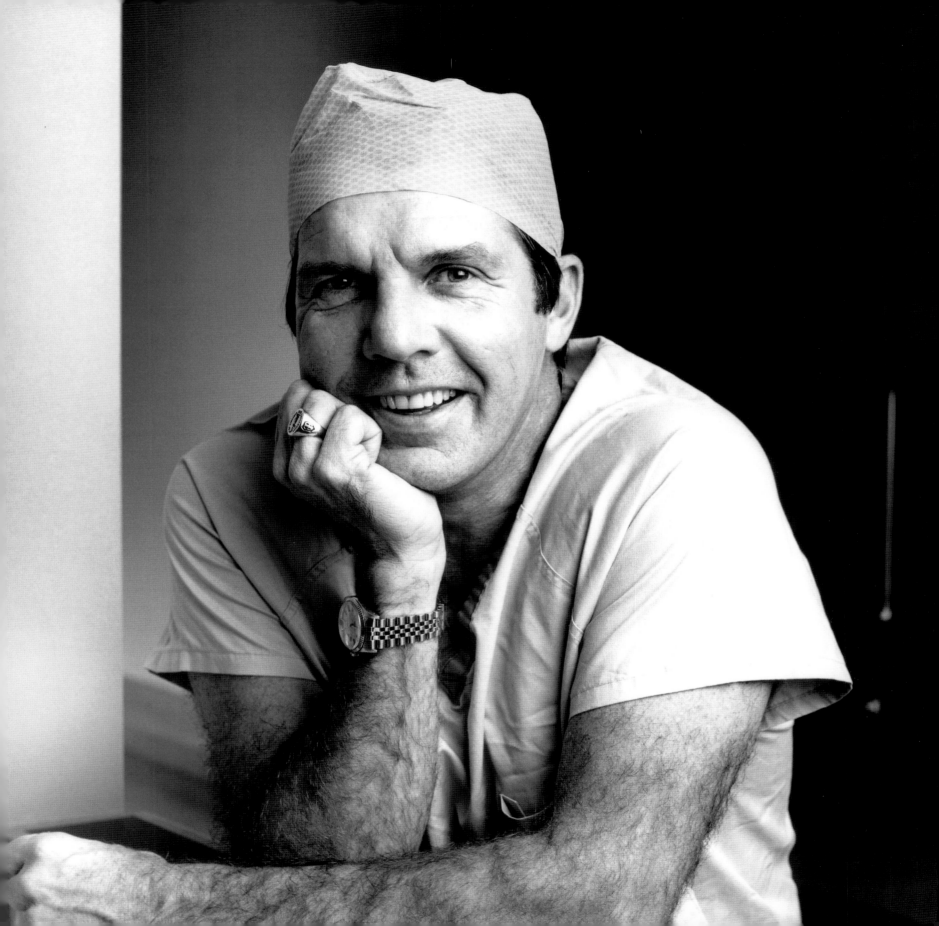

The Other Family Business

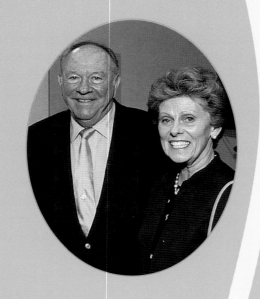

Harold Shepherd, the youngest of six children, was born on Oxford Road in Atlanta in 1928. When Harold was three, his father, William Clyde, moved the family out to LaVista Road, where his fledgling construction company would have more room for operations. LaVista was unpaved at the time, Harold remembers, "and between Briarcliff Road and what's now Toco Hills Shopping Center, there couldn't have been more than six houses."

On their 21-acre compound they had horses, pigs, chickens, a big vegetable garden, and, most important, more than a hundred mules — the heavy machinery of road-building at the time. "This was during the Depression," says Harold, "and how my daddy managed to feed a hundred mules and six children I'll never know." The Shepherd property later became, and remained for many years, the home of DeKalb Christian Academy.

Alana Smith, meanwhile, was spending her first thirteen years in Sioux City, Iowa, the daughter of a veterinarian who specialized in serum manufacturing. When her father's business brought the family to Atlanta, Alana enrolled at North Avenue Presbyterian School (NAPS), which would evolve into Westminster.

Harold and Alana became acquainted during their high school years (Harold went off to Darlington in Rome, Georgia and returned to graduate from Boys' High), and dated throughout Alana's years at Stephens College in Missouri. They were married at Druid Hills Presbyterian Church in 1949. That same year Harold joined older brothers Clyde and Dan in the family business, where all three are still active. "We've been in business together for fifty years," says Harold, "and we're still speaking."

Shepherd Construction Company's third-generation work force arrived in due course. James and his twin sister Dana were Harold and Alana's first children. Younger brother Tommy followed five years later. James and Tommy never considered working elsewhere. Along with their first cousins (Clyde's son, Clyde III, and Dan's son, Steve) James and Tommy now form the third generation executive corps of the parent company.

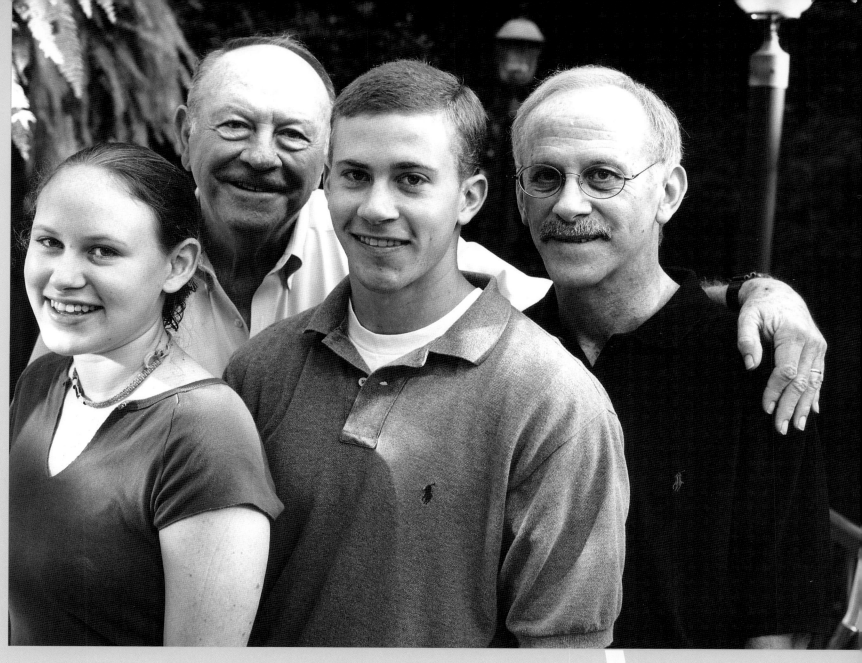

Three generations of Shepherds: Julie, Harold, Jamie, and James.

Nor does the family show any signs of relinquishing its hold on the business. James's son Jamie, a student at the University of Georgia, has already started working at the company during the summer, extending the dynasty into its fourth generation. Jamie's grandmother, for one, thinks the company will be in good hands: "He's a Hope Scholar and has made the Dean's List in the university's School of Business."

Early Years

Everybody remembers the space—or lack of it—at the leased Howell Mill Road facility . . . the one "gym," originally designed as a waiting area, maybe twenty-five feet by forty, where all the rehabilitation work with the patients took place—the floor mats, the elevated mats, the parallel bars, the pulleys, the standing table, the kitchen off to one side in a sort of alcove. "The gym was in the old entrance to the hospital," recalls Dr. Murray, "so people would still come up to the door and just walk through our area into the hospital, stepping over our patients who were lying on the floor."

But the chaos failed to impede what was an immediate and striking success. The snowball was rolling downhill, and the six-bed "demonstration project" quickly proved to the insurance industry, the medical community and the general population that a local spinal cord rehabilitation hospital would serve a tremendous need in and around Atlanta. "Within two weeks we had a waiting list," Alana Shepherd recalls. The six beds soon became twelve, and then twenty, as the two corridors leading off from the central area filled with spinal cord patients. "And by the time we got to twenty," Alana continues, "the waiting list had grown to forty."

Even with today's staff of more than eight hundred, Shepherd's close-knit family atmosphere remains a cherished value. Nevertheless, an occasional nostalgic twinge for a time when "everybody knew everybody" is certainly understandable. In those days the doctors were all called by their first names, just like the staff and patients. Alana remembers one patient who, in addition to his spinal cord injury, also had a brain injury—not debilitating, but enough so that he couldn't remember Dr. Murray's name and always called him "Herman Murphy" or, better yet, "Murph."

Growing out of the sense of intimacy and camaraderie was a very special relationship between the staff and the patients. "Because we were so small," says Joanie Ventresca, one of those three original therapists, "and because we were with the patients in the same room virtually all day long, we got very close. On our outings we did a lot of things you just can't do anymore, and the patients had a great time. Of course, our patients still go on wonderful outings, but . . . ." Montez Howard, who volunteered at the Howell Mill Road facility before joining the staff fulltime as a physical therapist, adds, "There just wasn't anything we wouldn't do for those patients."

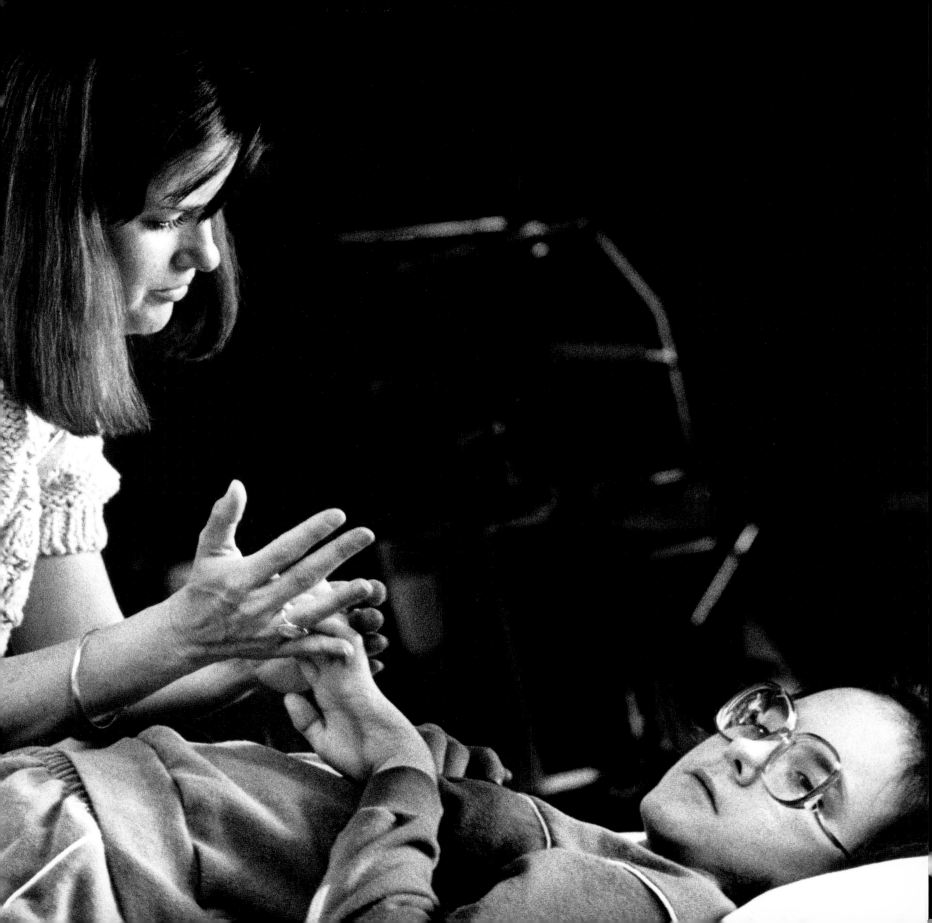

There was very little in the way of resources when I started. But there was a very strong vision, on the part of Alana and James and Dr. Apple, in terms of what they wanted. Without that very personal commitment on their part, I'm not sure we would have made it.

—Donna Smeltz
Director of Special Projects

Original Shepherd Center Staff

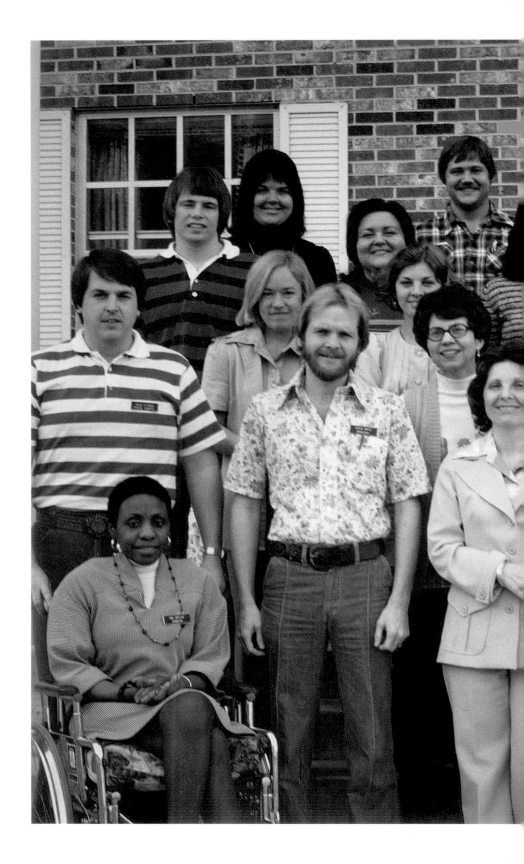

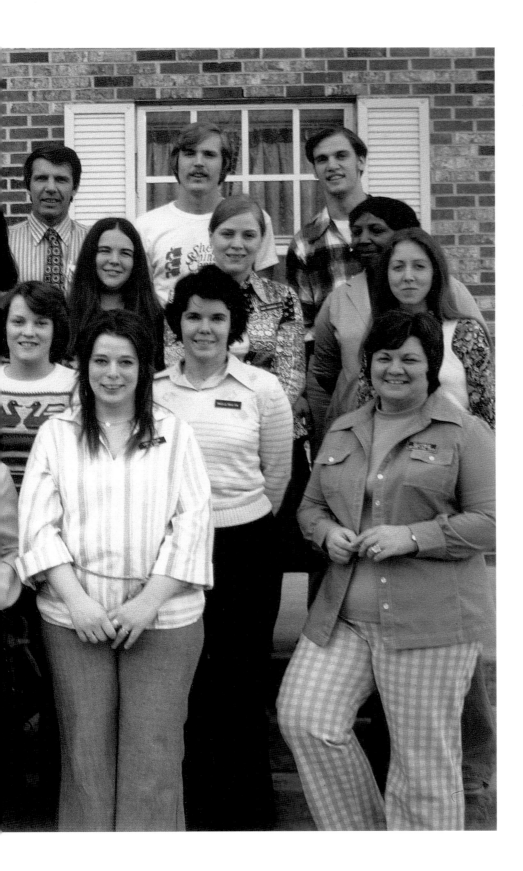

It was a pioneer spirit in the early days. The whole place had it, fostered it. I was encouraged and never stifled. I had incredible latitude in which to do my job.

—Lesley Hudson
Program Director,
Spinal Cord Injury
Model Systems Grant

13

Tammy King, who signed on as a medical assistant three days after the center opened and has remained on the staff ever since, recalls a vivid example of the prevailing attitude: "Patients didn't always have discharge plans, and I actually took a patient home with me once. Just threw a mattress on the floor, and she lived with me until she could figure out where she was going to go. Or we might put patients in our own cars to get them to school. This was the kind of thing we all did, because we just wanted so much to see them do better."

The staff also enjoyed in those early days an urgent and exhilarating sense of mission. "We were a youthful corps," recalls Lesley Hudson, who joined the center in early 1976 as its first administrator. "We felt like we were involved in something very special and extremely important. A pioneer spirit prevailed over the whole place." It wasn't for the traditionalist, the person who can function only in a structured environment. "In those days," says Lesley, "working here was either something you couldn't live without or couldn't get away from fast enough."

Montez, now the director of the spinal cord injury (SCI) program, echoes the sentiment: "What struck me was that nobody knew what we couldn't do. Now our roles are pretty clearly defined, but back then everybody did everything. We were just proceeding by trial and error, but our graduates were some of the best because we had such a close relationship with them." Donna Smeltz, who joined the nursing staff in 1979, adds that "the work was hard, very demanding, but what kept me excited and captivated was that sense of commitment from Dr. Apple and the Shepherds. We were involved in something very meaningful."

Lesley Hudson worked on whatever happened to get dropped on her desk, which she shared with Dr. Apple. Because it had originally been a patient room, their joint "office" had a connecting bathroom. In here Lesley laid an old door over the tub and created space for stacking her files. From the shower curtain rod hung the t-shirts that she was in charge of having printed up for the "graduates"—i.e., patients who were discharged. A small closet in the room housed the center's single copy machine.

"You had to be open to anything," says Lesley, "not sit there with a black line drawn around your job responsibilities. Out of that spirit came things like Field Day, graduation celebrations, holiday parties . . . it could get loud and raucous."

The great fun of those parties and celebrations also evokes many memories of the early years . . . of Dr. Apple in his red long johns, playing Santa at the first patients' Christmas party . . . of Dr. Bruce Green, Shepherd's original urologist, wailing on his saxophone . . . of wheelchair races and pie-eating contests at Field Day . . . of hilarious skits and "questionable talent" shows. Joanie

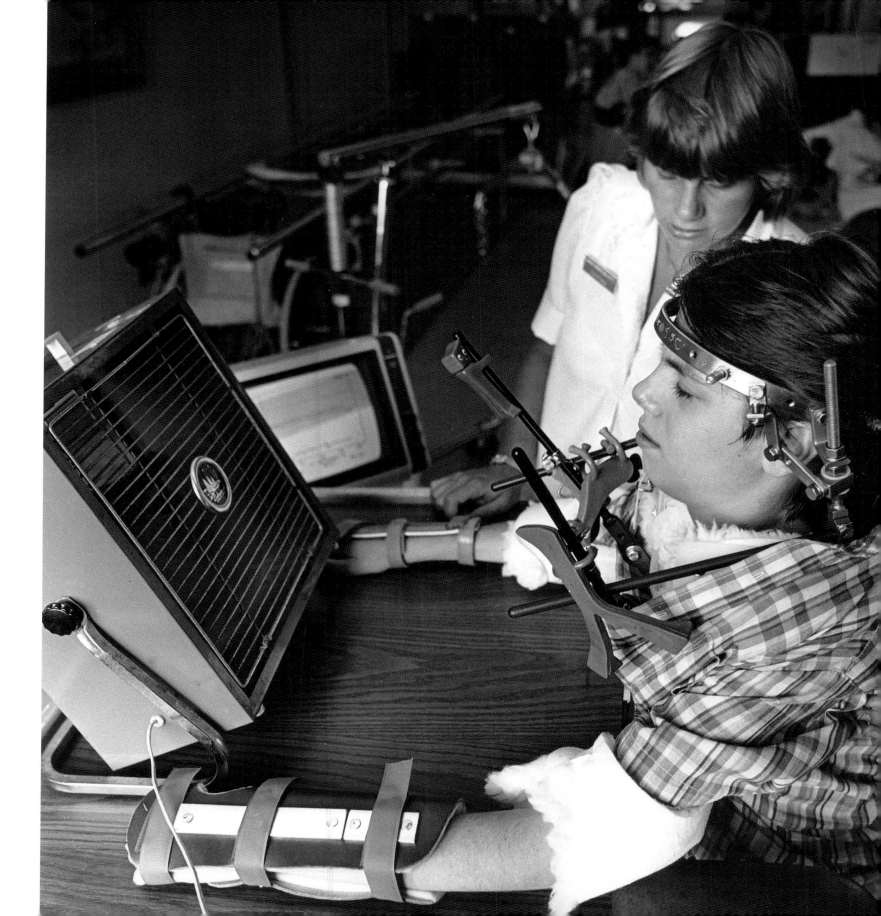

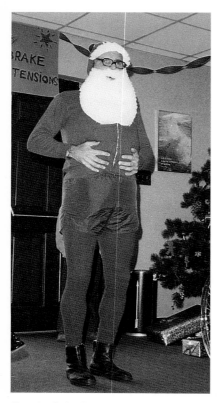

Dr. Apple in Santa costume

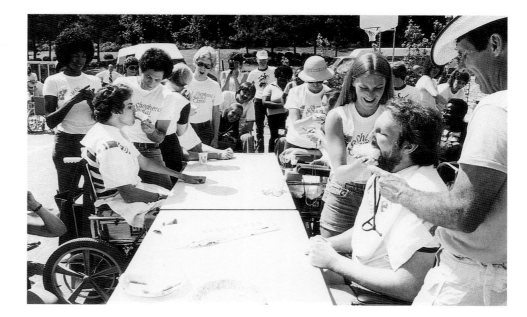

*Humor is definitely one of
our core values. For instance,
if you're thin-skinned or don't
want to be in the thick of
things, then steer clear of
our talent show.*

*—Gary R. Ulicny, Ph.D.
President and CEO*

Ventresca, along with Carol Coogler and Cathy Cox Shepherd—the other two original therapists—formed an ensemble known as the Dixie Cups, who specialized in outrageous parodies of then-current TV shows and movies. Alana remembers that in one of their skits they put a curly wig on Dr. Murray, had him lie down on his back on the floor of the gym, and spun him around like an upside-down turtle. "That kind of thing set the whole emotional tone for this place," she says, "where even the doctors are good enough sports to sacrifice their dignity to the delight of the patients."

And more than one original staffer remembers with special clarity the Halloween party featuring the "Happy Days" spoof, when Dave "The Fonz" Apple, piloting his motorcycle with Dr. Murray on the back, gunned the accelerator a bit harder than he intended, shot up the ramp, went airborne through the automatic doors, and landed with a long black skid-mark on the carpet inside the center. The expression of abject terror frozen on Dr. Murray's face, along with the death grip with which he clasped The Fonz, seem to have been similarly frozen in Shepherd Spinal Center's collective memory.

Indeed, since day one humor has always been a prized virtue at Shepherd. "Frankly," explains Joanie, "therapy itself can be pretty boring, and Carol's whole attitude was that we needed to make it as fun as we possibly could—and still get the work done." Montez Howard calls humor "one of our core values, and a tremendous help in our effort to deal with the most intimate details of our patients' lives."

Alana is less analytical: "Everybody was happy about being part of somebody's rehab; we were making people better. We laughed and joked a lot—still do."

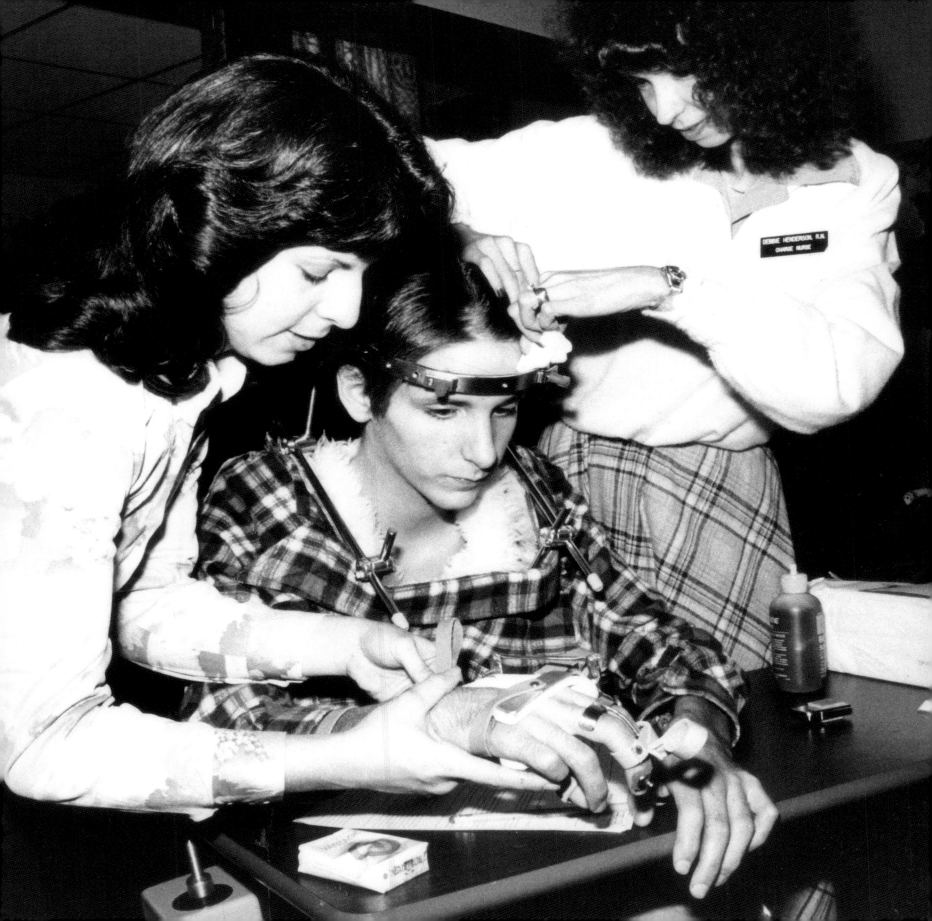

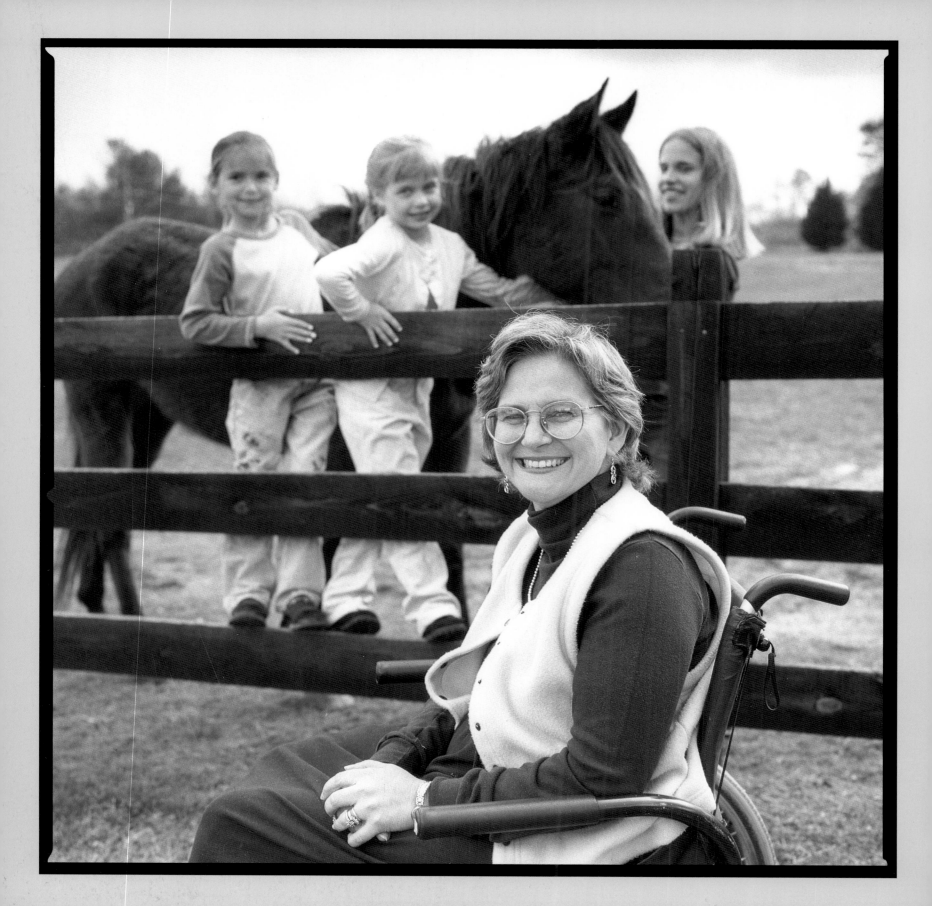

Paige Hawkins Martin

Paige Hawkins Martin is one of those special people whose life shines like a beacon. One of Shepherd Center's early patients, Paige was injured in 1976 at age 16, when the pickup truck she was riding in slipped off the road, flipped, and sent her flying through the windshield. She arrived at Shepherd from Athens General Hospital in a full body cast, but was discharged just two months later, ready to return to her sophomore year at Jefferson High. "I know my injury will not stop me from making my contribution," she said at the time.

In her senior year, Paige was elected class president, Miss Jefferson High School, and Homecoming Queen. She enrolled at Truett McConnell Junior College, and while working at a day care camp in Hall County, she realized that early childhood education would be her career. She attended Brenau College in Gainesville to complete her B.A. degree, and in 1986 received her Masters in Education. By this time Paige was already teaching second grade at Sardis Elementary in Gainesville.

She was also happily married — to Jerry Martin, an electrical engineer who drew up the plans, made blueprints, and, along with Paige's father, built the couple's "dream home" — wide hallways, huge bathrooms, custom-built kitchen cabinets — on five acres near Paige's school.

Today, Paige is still teaching at Sardis Elementary, but there have been a few changes along the way. Now, instead of second grade, she teaches kindergarten and first grade. "I took a year off to have my second child," Paige explains, "and when I went back the first grade position was available, so I've never gone back to second grade."

That's another change: Paige is the mother of two girls, a 12-year-old seventh grader and six-year-old first grader at Sardis.

And as for that dream home? "Well, actually," says Paige, "we've built a new home. The first one was great for three, but when we had our second child, we decided we needed more space. Inside and outside."

Paige elaborates: "When we built the second time, we moved back close to my parents, who have acreage, and we now have adjoining land and our pastures back up to each other. So there's plenty of room for our three horses and our mule. We also have a dog, two cats, and some fish, and the animals on the inside of the house are a lot more trouble than the animals on the outside."

When Paige and Jerry are not chauffeuring the girls to basketball, softball, gymnastics and cheerleading, they are likely to be volunteering at church. Paige has taught Sunday School classes in the past, and she and Jerry remain constantly involved in church committee work.

How the years have flown by for Paige, who was a patient when Shepherd was one year old. "It's funny," she reflects, "My youngest daughter has never been to Shepherd. I'll have to take her one of these days, so she can see what that's all about."

(Thanks to Marty Church's profile of Paige, "Where Are They Now?" in Spinal Column, September 1986, p. 8.)

> "My youngest daughter has never been to Shepherd. I'll have to take her one of these days, so she can see what that's all about."

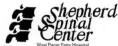

Shepherd Spinal Center

West Paces Ferry Hospital

3200 Howell Mill Road, N.W.   Atlanta, Georgia 30327   Telephone: 351-0351

VOL. 2 • SPRING 1978 | QUARTERLY NEWSLETTER

FROM THE DESK OF THE MEDICAL DIRECTOR:

In 1975, when the Shepherd Spinal Center opened with six beds, it was the projection of the hospital that the average occupancy during the first year would be approximately seven patients. However, by the end of the first year, the number of beds had expanded to twenty, and these beds were continuously full with a long waiting list. The need for a spinal care facility had definitely been demonstrated.

During the last year and a half of operation, it has been necessary to expand the spinal center capacity by opening a Skin Care Unit within the West Paces Ferry Hospital to accomodate six additional patients. Last month, that unit was relocated and it is now in the same building with the spinal center. Additionally, spinal cord injured patients with medical problems are admitted to the acute portion of West Paces Ferry Hospital whenever overflow beds are needed.

A recent review of our statistics for all spinal cord injured patients, compiled over the past twenty-seven months, indicated that a forty bed hospital would be both a financially sound and medically necessary plan for the immediate future.

With this record of growth, and after a review of the appropriate statistics, it has been determined that the Shepherd Spinal Center needs larger quarters. At this time an active effort is being formulated to bring an enlarged Shepherd Spinal Center into reality. The enlargement will not only encompass the ability to handle more patients on an in-patient basis, but will be directed towards enlarging the capabilities of the out-patient clinic. It is envisioned that the latter not only will take care of the routine follow-up, but will provide a better setting for the diagnosis of general health conditions, including dental care.

The next twelve months will constitute an exciting era in the growth and development of the Shepherd Spinal Center as a full scale treatment facility for all problems dealing with spinal cord injury. As progress is made, it is our intention to keep you posted in order to promote your continued interest and allow you to share in our progress and expansion.

David F. Apple, Jr., M.D.
Medical Director

Pat Latham, R.N.
Department Manager

Growing Pains

When the first issue of the "Quarterly Newsletter" appeared in the fall of 1977, Shepherd Spinal Center had been in operation for two years and had admitted more than two hundred patients for an average length of stay of 59 days. Such numbers were sufficient to lay to rest forever any question of the center's viability, but they also portended conflict with the landlord.

"It was never a good arrangement," says Alana. "For one thing, we were a not-for-profit charitable organization in a for-profit hospital. And then when we began putting our patients in other parts of the hospital, it seemed to cause them problems."

"It was fine when that space had been empty," explains Dr. Apple, who as medical director stood in the line of fire. "But once the hospital started filling up with its own patients, we began pinching their bottom line. They didn't have a lot of motivation to take on our long-staying, low-volume clientele. They could bring in more revenue by removing tonsils."

Although, in Dr. Apple's words, "we had to beg, borrow, and steal to make any improvements in the program," improvements nevertheless continued steadily. In January 1978, the addition of a third registered nurse (R.N.) position made possible the initiation of the long-anticipated outpatient program. Directed by Kathy McKee, the program instituted routine follow-up visits with every patient within three to six months after discharge, giving patients and their families the opportunity to discuss questions and problems about their continuing at-home rehabilitation and, importantly, reducing the number of costly hospital readmissions. The program also constituted an invaluable source of patient information to the center's growing research effort.

One month later, another pressing need was addressed when the center opened a six-bed skin care unit under the supervision of Armide Price, R.N. The immobility associated with spinal cord injury can result in skin ulcerations, which in themselves can cause serious, and costly, medical complications. The new unit offered special nursing attention to patients with such problems, as well as an educational program for patients and their families designed to help prevent recurrence.

Shortly after the skin unit opened, Dr. Apple used his column in the newsletter to voice what was quickly becoming the consensus opinion: "A recent review of our statistics for all spinal cord injured patients, compiled over the past twenty-seven months, indicates that a forty-bed hospital would be both a financially sound and medically necessary plan for the immediate future."

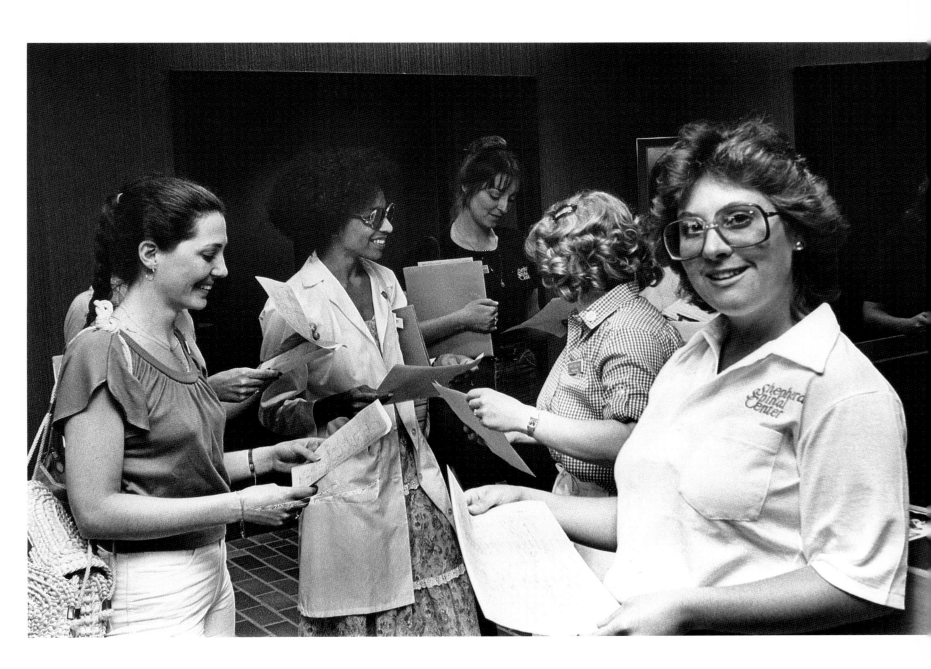

Shepherd's own facility did lie in the future, but that future was perhaps not as "immediate" as Dr. Apple and his staff would have liked. In the meantime, growth was unabated. Whereas total admissions after two years numbered 211, after a third year that number had nearly doubled, to 417. The outpatient clinic was recording equally impressive statistics. By November—still in its first year of operation—between 15 and 20 patients were being treated in the clinic every Wednesday—its designated day of business.

And in January 1979, yet another program was added, one that would eventually become a hallmark of Shepherd's excellence in total rehabilitative care: therapeutic recreation (see story, p. 107). The hiring of Barb Leidheiser as Shepherd's first recreation therapist fulfilled the special wish of both James Shepherd and Dr. Apple. James could vividly remember his own rehabilitation at Craig Hospital and how desperately he wanted to "do something fun." In fact, he got "grounded" for sneaking off to ride a three-wheeler (all-terrain vehicle) while wearing his neck brace. As for Dr. Apple, his work made it obvious that injured people still need recreation, "and if you could get them to thinking about going back to fishing or hunting, then it's a logical transition from there to even more important things, like becoming a mom or dad or going back to school or work."

Needless to say, the hospital failed to see this need and refused to fund the position. Until the hospital administration finally came around, Barb Leidheiser's compensation came directly out of Dr. Apple's pocket. And the program's first van—an absolute necessity for patient outings—was a gift of the Shepherd (Family) Foundation.

Continuing its steady expansion, by the time it celebrated its fourth anniversary in the summer of '79, the center employed 60 full-time staffers and boasted a "comprehensive program" of spinal cord injury rehabilitation: acute stabilization and transportation to the center; evaluation; intensive nursing and therapy programs; education of patient and family; equipment prescription and purchase; driver evaluation and vehicle modification; psychological and aptitude testing and vocational counseling; home, workplace, and school accessibility evaluations; and final discharge planning. It was also a matter of pride that Shepherd's was the only such program in the state of Georgia. "Of course, that was one of the reasons we grew so rapidly," says Dr. Murray. "The other hospitals in Georgia badly needed a place to send spinal cord injured patients, and early on we gained their confidence and trust in the job we were doing."

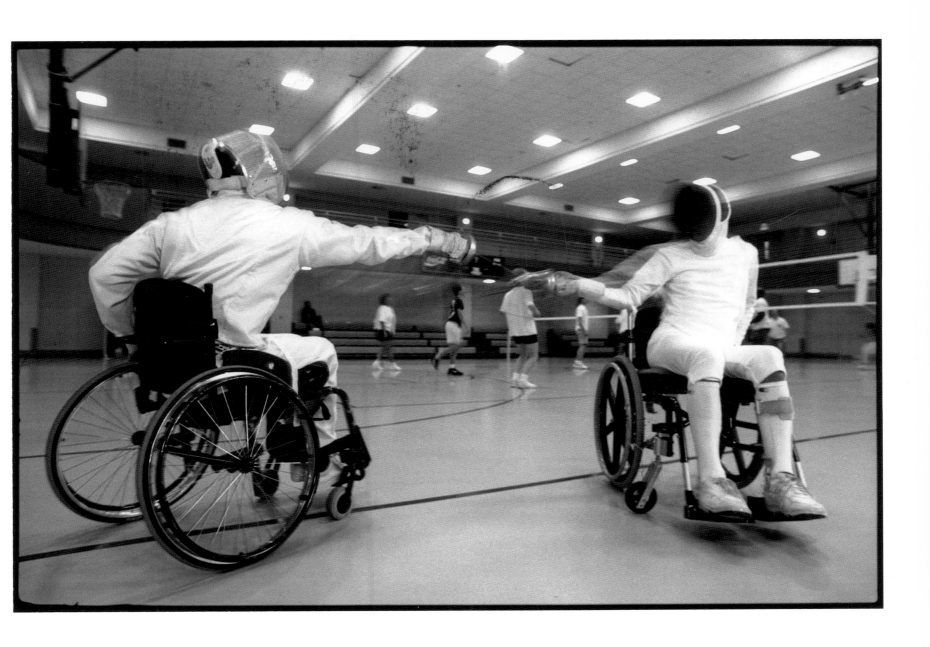

Concrete Dreams

But even before its fourth birthday party, the big news was announced. Shepherd Spinal Center would construct its own facility on Peachtree Road just north of Piedmont Hospital. It was the ideal location, but securing the site, as Alana remembers, had required an enormous behind-the-scenes effort. "Based on their philosophy that moving into an existing facility would be more cost effective, the State of Georgia health planning system made us investigate all the Atlanta area hospitals for space. Emory's new Rehabilitation and Therapy Center offered us 20 beds, but we knew we would eventually want 80 beds, the number Craig has. St. Joseph offered us free land, but we would have been encircled by the expressway and would have had no amenities for our patients. It went on and on."

As it happened, Atlanta developer Scott Hudgens had the property on Peachtree Road for sale. "Piedmont Hospital was interested in buying it," remembers Alana; "McDonald's wanted to buy it, but Scott and his wife Jackie wanted to see the property used for a special purpose. Harold and Scott were old friends, and Scott knew all about what we were doing with Shepherd Spinal Center, so he ultimately decided to sell us the property for $1 million. He also extended the option, when we weren't able to raise the money as fast as we said we would, and once we had raised the money and were ready to close, in the elevator on the way to the closing Scott handed James a check, a personal gift, for $200,000. So, in effect, we got the perfect piece of property for $800,000—a fabulous price."

Along with the announcement—in the summer of '79—came architect's renderings of the proposed building and, of course, a major fundraising initiative. At the board of directors' October meeting, Barge Construction Company was selected as the general contracting firm for the new facility, with groundbreaking scheduled for late spring, 1980. Henry Smith would be the architect for the project, bringing his tenure on the board of directors to an abrupt end. As Smith recalls, "Frank Carter came to me and said, 'You can't be the architect and be on the board. That would be a conflict of interest.' I said, 'Frank, I've just resigned from the board.'"

Also in October, the boards of Piedmont Hospital and its Foundation hosted the Shepherd board at the Piedmont Driving Club. The Piedmont

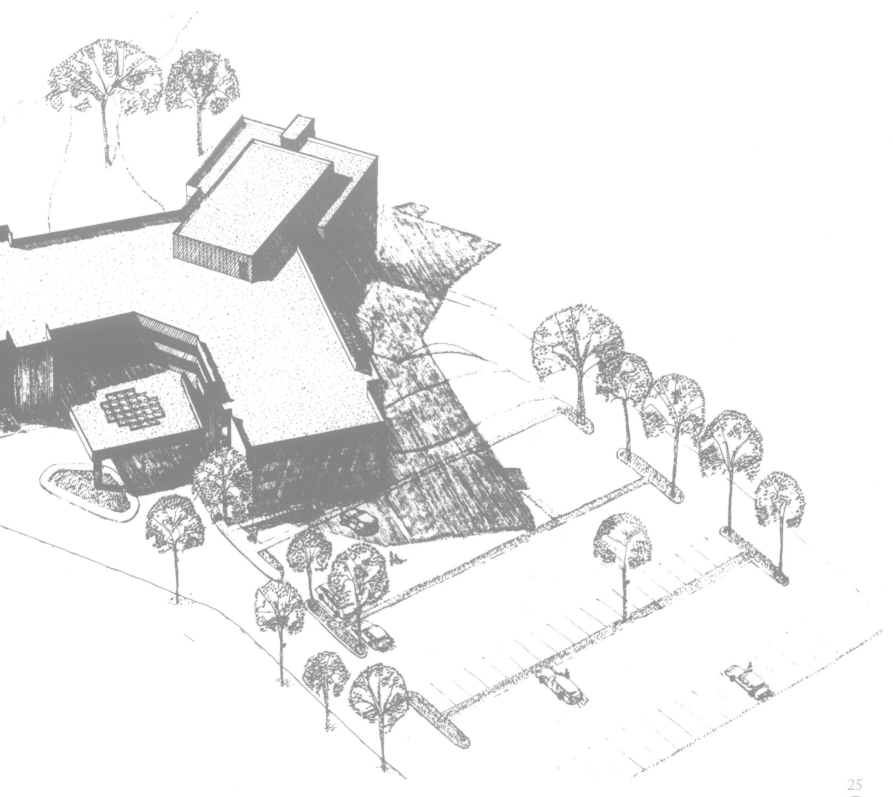

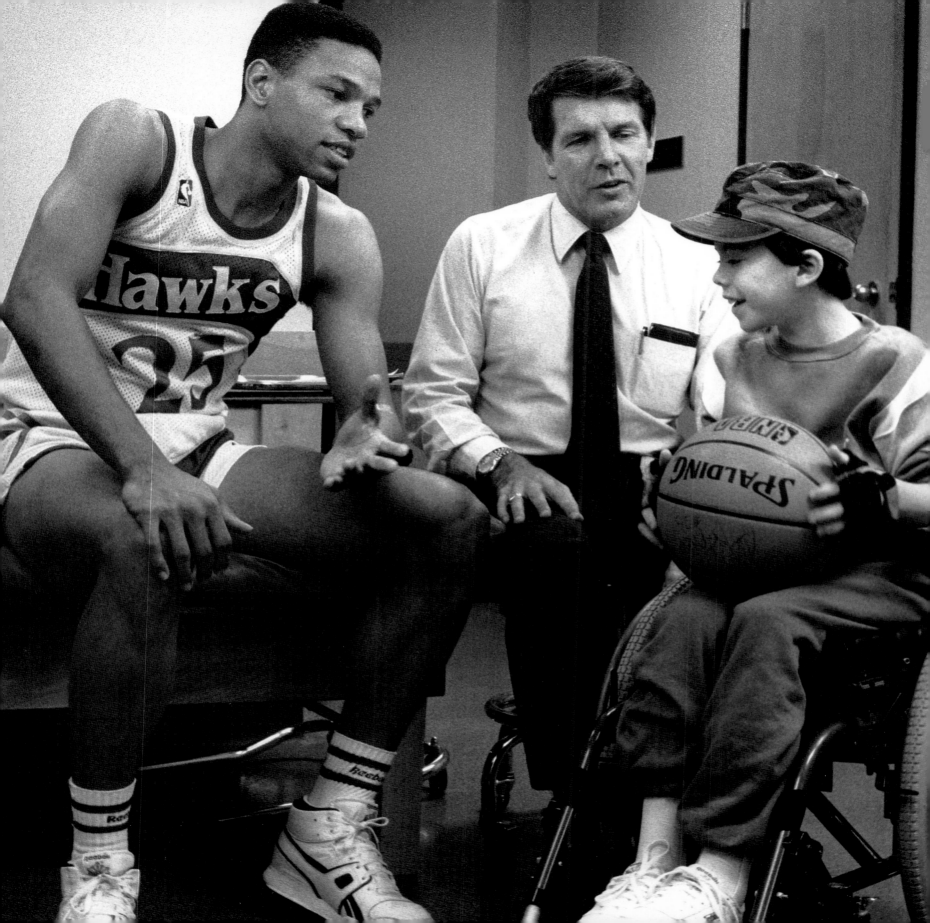

Hospital and Foundation trustees took the opportunity to extend their welcome and to express the eagerness of the entire Piedmont community to have Shepherd Spinal Center as a neighbor.

By March 1, 1980, $3 million had been raised—out of a projected total of $5 million. A gift from the Samuel Roberts Noble Foundation of $250,000 gave the fundraising effort a welcome shot of adrenaline. Meanwhile, excitement was rapidly building in anticipation of the features to be included in the new facility's 93,000 square feet of space:

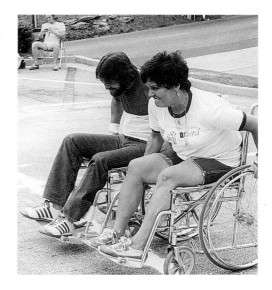

- forty beds immediately, with built-in capacity to expand to eighty;
- intensive care beds on the nursing unit, so patients would have continuous care from injury through discharge at the same location;
- radiology, laboratory, and pharmacy units;
- a comprehensive, full-time outpatient clinic;
- and a patient apartment to help patients nearing discharge make the transition to independent living.

The services to be provided through Piedmont Hospital—operating rooms, housekeeping, food services, and others—would be rendered with the convenience of a corridor connecting the two hospitals.

Amid this frenzy of anticipation, Shepherd Spinal Center neared its fifth birthday, marked by the celebration of the biggest and best Field Day yet. More than a hundred people were on hand for a full slate of hotly contested events, beginning with the "Three-Wheel Race" (two wheelchairs strapped together, with a doctor in one and a patient in another), and followed by the basketball toss and pie eating contests. The perennial patient favorite, Squirt the Staff, that year evolved into a dunk-fest, thanks to the rental of a "Dunk 'Em Machine" from a local carnival. Patients who could throw dunked their selected staffer by the traditional means. Others tied the platform lever to their chairs and dunked 'em by simply driving away. "Mean Bruce Green," after five years of futility, finally won the Doctors' Relay (wherein the docs negotiate an obstacle course while hampered by back, neck, and leg braces). Guest appearances by the Atlanta Hawks' "Tree" Rollins and sports columnist Furman Bisher lent a celebrity luster to the event.

Breaking Ground

But as summer turned to fall, Shepherd Spinal Center's collective attention focused on 2020 Peachtree Road, where, on the beautiful, crisp morning of October 13, 1980, a dozen ceremonial shovels broke the ground to officially initiate the construction of the new facility. "It was essential that we have our own

campus and control our own destiny," says James, "and that ceremony was a wonderful sign that it was really happening." Construction of the building was projected at fourteen months, with the move-in slated for January 1982.

The groundbreaking also kicked off the final phase of fundraising, which was
given a huge boost by Dottie and J. B. Fuqua's gift of $600,000, the largest single
donation to date. At the same time, however, Dr. Apple was using his forum in
Spinal Column, the center's quarterly magazine, to encourage donors to dig deep; a
$1.5 million "shortfall" would have to be covered if the hospital was to be debt-free.

By early spring of 1981, the building's first-story floor had been laid, and
progress continued steadily throughout the summer and fall. By the end of
September the building was "dried in"—meaning that the coming winter's
weather would be no hindrance. The projected move-in date was pushed to early
March, 1982.

In the meantime, a different kind of work was being carried on "off campus," the vital importance of which would only be measured as the years passed.
The Shepherd Spinal Center Auxiliary was incorporating its charter and elect-
ing its first officers, as follows:

- Gracie Schwartzman, President;
- Sara Shadburn (Chapman), Secretary;
- Jane Duggan, Treasurer;
- Carol Lanier Goodman, Membership Chairman;
- Marian Stevens, Chair of Volunteer Services;
- Anne DeBorde, Board of Directors Liaison; and
- Katharine Jones, Advisory Board Liaison.

These early volunteers, and those they recruited, would come to play a
tremendous part in the continuing growth and success of the hospital.

As the year ended, the total price tag for the new facility had grown to $8
million, and the projected shortfall to $2.6 million. Clearly, the center would
have to borrow money to complete the construction of the new facility. The good
news was that the necessary money would be available . . . and at a favorable
interest rate. Back in October, the Fulton County Hospital Authority had signed
a $3.5 million bond issue, which was bought by Trust Company Bank.

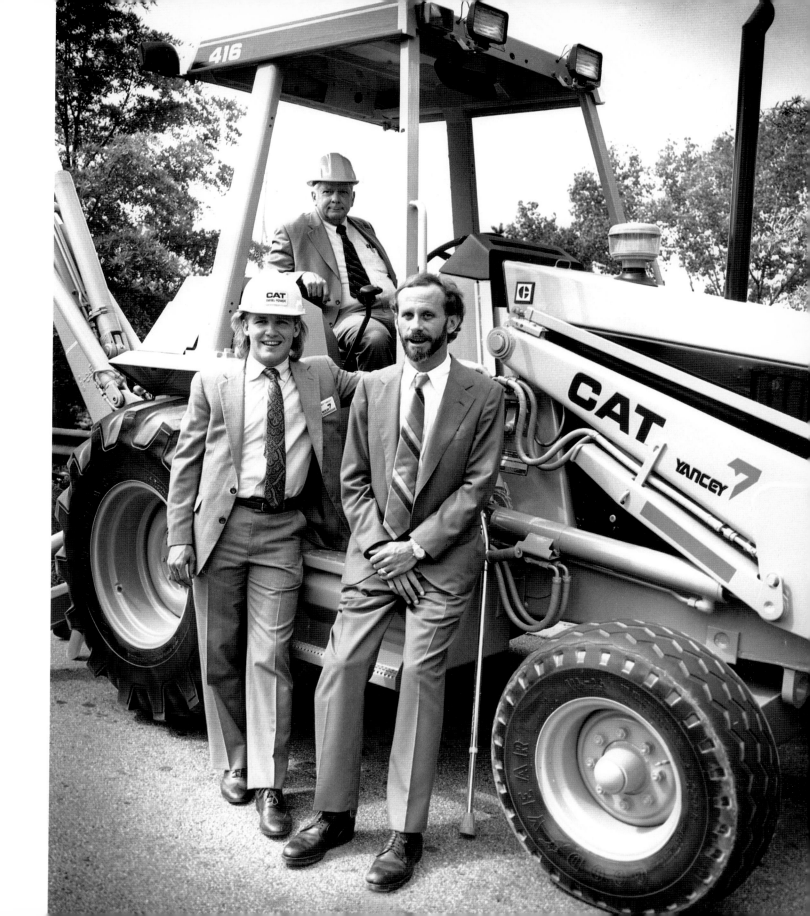

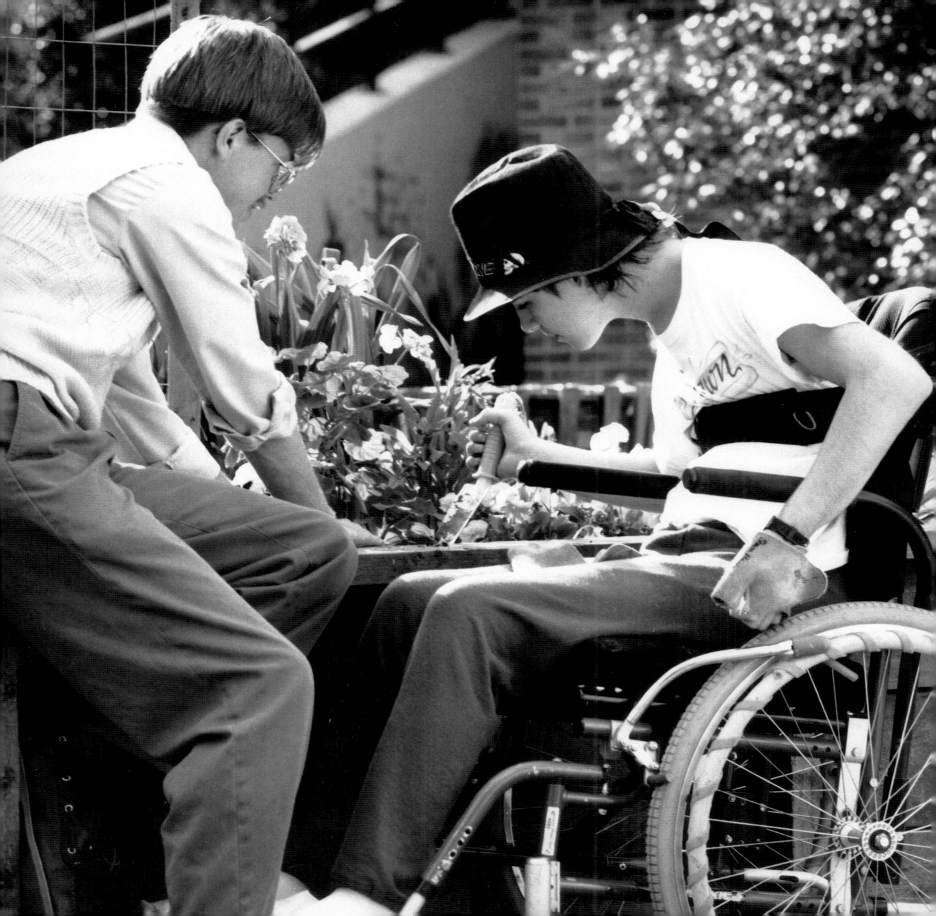

Auxiliary? Necessity!

"We did everything," says Sara Chapman, remembering the days back before the move to Peachtree Road when the "Auxiliary," informal and unchartered, consisted of a handful of volunteers. "Back then Shepherd really had hardly any staff, so everything that wasn't a matter of doctors, nurses, and therapists, we did."

Sara is not likely to forget her original "fundraising" effort for the Auxiliary. With Shepherd as the designated beneficiary of all the money thrown into the fountain at Lenox Square Mall, it was Sara's job to raise the funds, by hand, right out of the drained fountain pools. "I'd bag all these coins—slimy dimes and nickels and pennies—drop them in the trunk of my car (probably wearing out my axles), take them home, clean and roll up all the coins, and take them to the bank. I'm talking maybe several thousand dollars at a time."

With the impending move to the new facility, the time was right to formally incorporate the organization. "A small group of us," says Sara, "Gracie Schwartzman, Carol Goodman, Anne DeBorde, Marian Stevens, Kay Jones, Jane Duggan, and I started meeting extensively with Alana to formalize the organization, with by-laws, a charter, the whole thing. Board member and attorney Ted Forbes wrote the by-laws for us. Then we sent out, on our stationery, with our logo, five hundred letters inviting people to join the organization. Out of that membership drive came the original Life Members, and we were officially off and running."

In those days the Auxiliary was literally a "helping" organization, with emphasis on relieving the overburdened and undermanned hospital staff. "'Whatever it takes' was our motto," says Sara, "and we were very hands-on." Working with the patients was an integral part of their mission—patient care, feeding, outings, entertainment, games, running the gift shop . . . even helping with mat exercises.

It was demanding work, and very rewarding. In fact, seeing volunteers like Laura Smith actually helping the patients with their exercises is one of Alana's fondest memories from the early days. "These people would actually be behind the patients on the table, helping hold them up, helping them work on their range of motion. Imagine what a wonderful experience it was for those volunteers. I know that many of them have never forgotten it."

Over the years, fundraising has become an important function of the Auxiliary as well. Pecans on Peachtree, the Southeastern Charity Horse Show (for twelve years, or as long as Sara handled the production of the show's 120-page program) and, the Legendary Party (since its inaugural in 1989) have been spectacularly successful Auxiliary fundraisers. In fact, in recent years, the annual total of the monies raised by the organization has exceeded a half million dollars.

At right are the names of the generous and spirited ladies who have served as the Auxiliary's president since its inception almost twenty years ago:

1982-83: Gracie Schwartzman

1983-84: Marian Stevens

1984-85: Sara Chapman

1985-86 and 1986-87: Audrey Bridell

1987-88: Ada Lamon

1988-89: Ann Carter McDonald

1989-90: Jane Duggan

1990-91: Carole Halverson

1991-92: Peggy Schwall

1992-93: Jane Gibson

1993-94: Claire Smith

1994-95: Sandra Flint

1995-96: Lynn Poole

1996-97: Marnite Calder

1997-98: Cookie Aftergut

1998-99: Lora Gray

1999-2000 and 2000-01: Lois Puckett

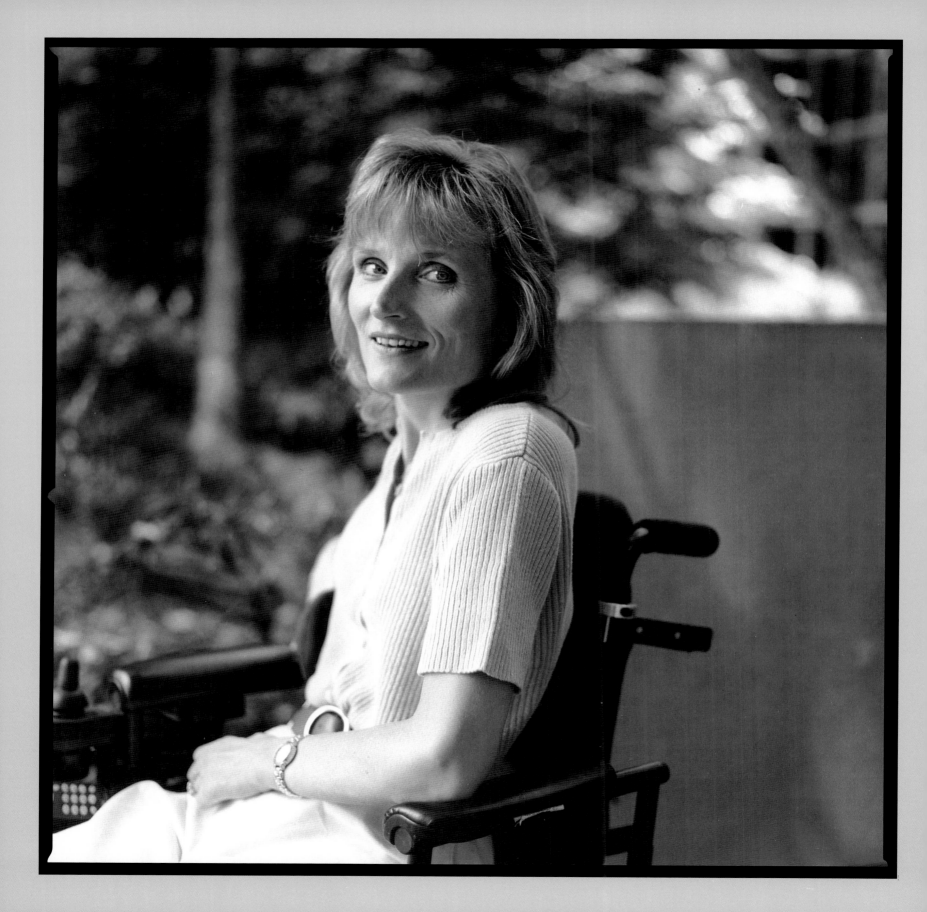

On the evening of September 10, 1980, Madge Pentecost was on her way to enroll at Young Harris College in northwest Georgia. As she rounded a curve close to Dahlonega, her car tipped over onto the driver's side and slid off the road.

Her neck was broken, but at first she didn't realize the gravity of her injury. Ironically, her father had broken his neck the previous year, but had been paralyzed for only a matter of hours. Madge was confident that she, too, would be all right in an hour or two.

But the headlights went out when her car turned over, and Madge lay in the dark until after midnight. Passers-by could not hear her cries for help, and eventually she felt herself lapsing into shock.

When at last a couple noticed the overturned vehicle and stopped to help, Madge was taken by ambulance to Lumpkin County Hospital, then transported to Gainesville General Hospital. Gainesville General sent her on to Kennestone Hospital in Marietta, where she lay in traction for eight days. She was transferred to Shepherd Spinal Center on September 19, and two days later Dr. David Apple performed a fusion. He removed bone chips and fragments from around the break and wired a good vertebra to the injured one. Nine weeks later Madge was discharged, just in time to spend Thanksgiving with her family.

Then, having missed scarcely a beat, Madge was back in school. She enrolled at Georgia State in January 1981 and graduated Cum Laude in March of 1984. She interviewed with several companies during her last quarter in school, but one in particular — Management Science America — caught her eye.

"On the day of my last exam at GSU, MSA notified me that I had the job," Madge recalls. "Back then MSA had 2,500 employees worldwide, and as far as I knew I was the only one in a wheelchair."

In the early '90s, MSA was bought out by Dunn & Bradstreet Software, and Madge stayed with the new company until it, in turn, was bought out in 1997. Since then she's been with Indus International, a developer of Enterprise Asset Management systems, where she manages a technical support team.

This dedicated career woman nevertheless finds plenty of time for community service. After taking the spotlight as Miss Wheelchair Georgia in 1986, Madge has become a spokesperson for such issues as seat belt safety, canine assistance, and disability awareness. She also teaches a Bible Study class at her church.

And Madge feels she has even more to offer. "For example," she says, "since my injury I have traveled a whole lot, especially for business. I would like to figure out a way to share what I have learned and become a resource for disabled travelers."

If it was not full enough already, a wonderful new dimension was added to Madge's life on September 9, 2000, when she was married to Brent Williams, an instructor in Kennesaw State University's instructional technology department.

In fact, Madge acknowledges, gratefully, that her success and achievements send a wonderful message. "In addition to the care and encouragement I got at Shepherd," she says, "my mother and father were tremendously supportive. Now, though, both my parents have passed away, and here I am. I have my own home, I have a good job, I have a new marriage, I manage my own life financially. I mean, I'm really independent.

"What my life shows people, I think," she concludes, "is that you are still able to go on."

(Spinal Column originally profiled Madge in July 1984, p. 12)

Madge Pentecost

"What my life shows people, I think, is that you are still able to go on."

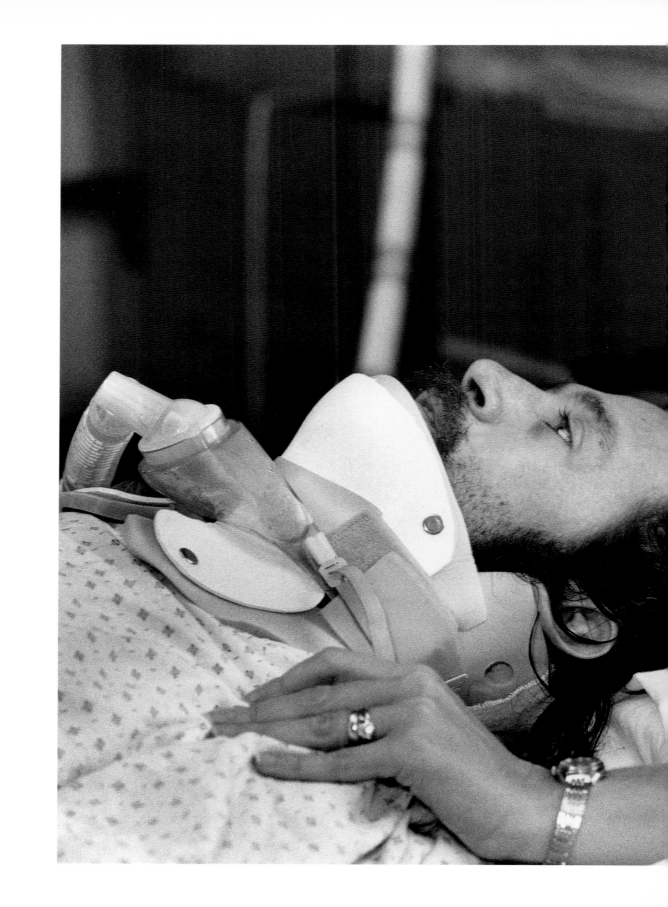

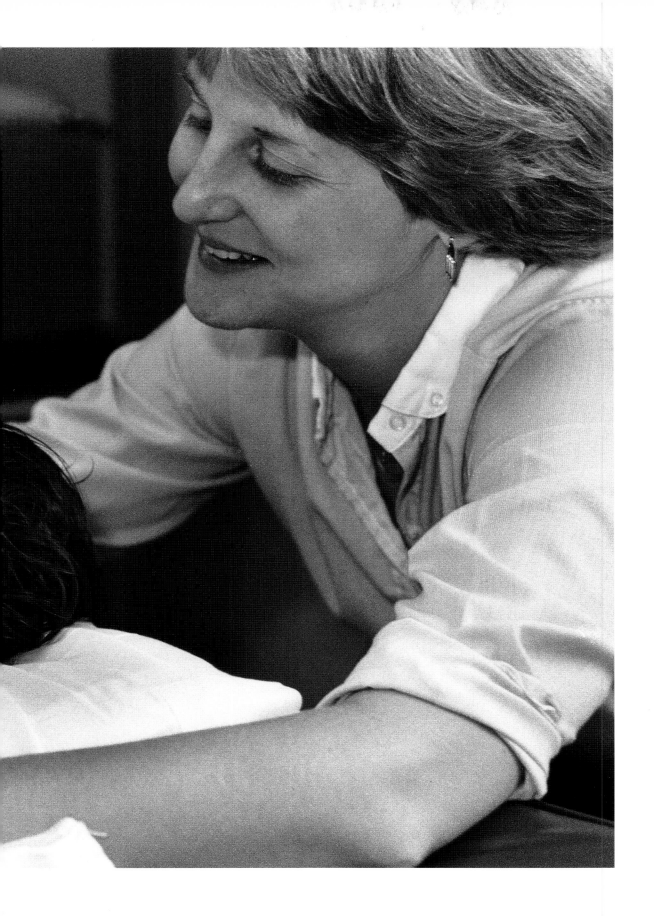

With the grand opening ceremonies set for April 22 (not much later, after all, than the original projections) the early months of 1982 were a blur of activity and anticipation. In the rush to complete floorings and fixtures, considerable attention was also being given to aesthetic amenities. Renowned weavers Susan Starr and Ken Weaver were commissioned to create decorative wall hangings, while photographer Renata Levy was conceptualizing her "Patients in Action" project—a series of photos illustrating what could be accomplished by the spinal cord injured who were treated at Shepherd Spinal Center.

Meanwhile, in one of those wonderful coincidences that seem to occur in the service of good, the father of Carol Coogler, the center's original chief physical therapist, happened to be C. S. "Bo" Coogler, the owner of a monument wholesale business in Elberton, Georgia. Because of his daughter's dedication to the work of the center, Mr. Coogler offered to provide the street marker to adorn the entrance to the hospital. No small contribution: the marker—made from the finest Georgia granite and including the name, original logo, and the street number—was nine feet long, four feet high, and weighed eight and a half tons.

Yet further removed from the building site, one more craftsman's work was being unveiled. In March, at the Piedmont Driving Club, where the Kappa Kappa Gamma Sorority was sponsoring its annual "Fashions and Diamonds Luncheon"—which, by the way, raised $7,500 to furnish a patient room in the new facility—the Shepherd "Angel" was introduced by local KKG chapter president Linda Clements. Quickly embraced as a way to express gratitude for volunteer service, the annual Angel Luncheon has become one of Shepherd's cherished traditions.

With the patient census reduced to six (to facilitate the move insofar as was possible) and with a staff recruitment campaign in full swing, the appointed day at last arrived. Eight hundred guests—board and advisory board members, staff, former patients, and contributors to the fundraising effort—were on hand to watch the ceremonial ribbon-cutting, performed by five of the men who turned the first shovels of dirt at the groundbreaking: former patients (and advisory board members) Martin Marchman and Judge Greeley Ellis, along with board members David Webb, Clark Harrison, and James Shepherd.

It was a festive occasion . . . and a tremendously significant one. Long-awaited and anxiously anticipated, Shepherd Spinal Center at 2020 Peachtree Road, free-standing, unbeholden, and in command of its own fate, was at last a reality. James Shepherd, for one, remembers the dedication ceremony as perhaps his single favorite moment in the center's history: "I'll never forget seeing founding board member Dave Webb lean over in his wheelchair to cut the ribbon. Tears were streaming down his face . . . and I knew that his feelings mirrored

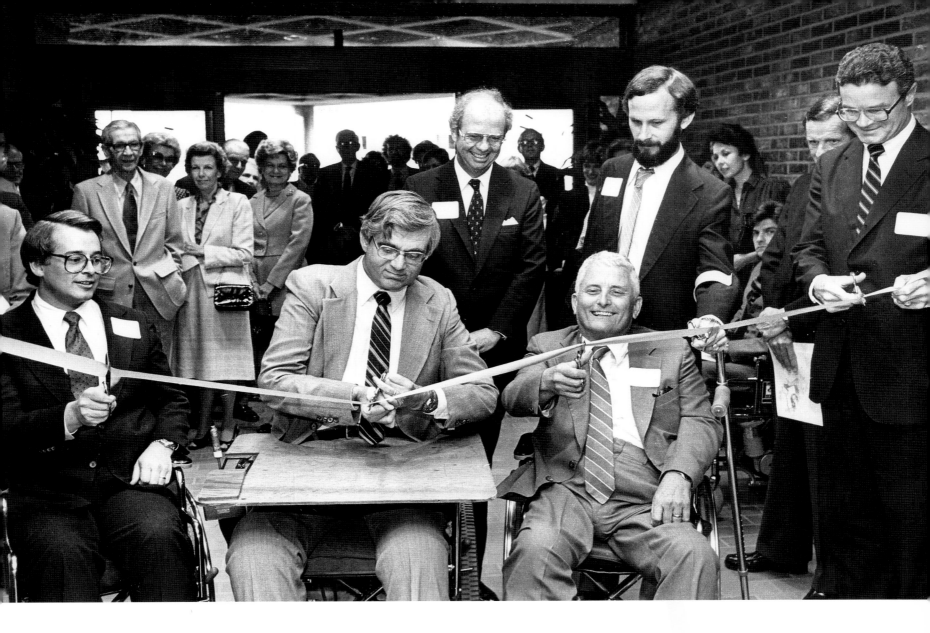

mine exactly. This great man, who had done more and experienced more than I had in my own lifetime, was literally weeping with joy. It was then I realized we really were a success. We had arrived."

"It was grand and glorious," adds Alana.

"Totally exhilarating," declares Dr. Apple. "Sure, we had some procedural things to work out, but even that had its own excitement. For me, it was pure liberation."

The Day After . . .

About those "procedural things." "It was pretty scary," recalls Donna Smeltz. "At the old facility, for all its shortcomings, we had an infrastructure and procedures in place. When we first opened here, we had none of that, no guidelines in place with Piedmont, so every time something new came up, it was 'Oh, damn, what do we do now?' The first couple of nights, Dave [Apple] spent the night here, and for a while we came in on weekends, just to make sure that the systems were working.

"And at the same time we still had these six patients that had made the move with us. Their rehab and medical needs had to be met while we were trying to figure out all this other stuff. I don't remember ever being so stressed in my life."

Those six patients were a problem for the board of directors, too—though for a diametrically opposite reason. "We had intentionally gotten our patient roster down to six to make the move," recalls Harold Shepherd, "so now all of a sudden we're sitting there looking at that huge building, those 40 beds, and thinking, 'How are we gonna pay for this thing?'"

But as Dr. Apple is quick to point out, "Whatever initial adjustment problems we may have had, those six patients were a whole lot better off than they ever were on Howell Mill Road, and that's the bottom line." Furthermore, as for the worries of the board, the number didn't hold at six for very long. Within a very few weeks—in fact, as quickly as the necessary staff could be recruited and trained— the patient roster climbed to its maximum of 40.

Among those recent recruits was a valuable addition to Dr. Apple's medical staff: Dr. Allen P. McDonald, who had been "helping out" at Shepherd for several years before officially coming on board a few months prior to the move to Peachtree Road. A native Atlantan, Dr. McDonald had developed a keen interest in the treatment of spinal fracture during his residency and subsequently did a fellowship in spinal cord injury at Rancho Los Amigos in California. Now a partner – along with Dr. Herndon Murray – of Peachtree Orthopedic Clinic, Dr. McDonald approaches his 20th year as one of Shepherd's attending physicians. "What continues to motivate me in my work at Shepherd," says Dr. McDonald, "is the chance to have something positive to offer patients with debilitating injuries. They often think it's the end of the world, and we help them see that it's not."

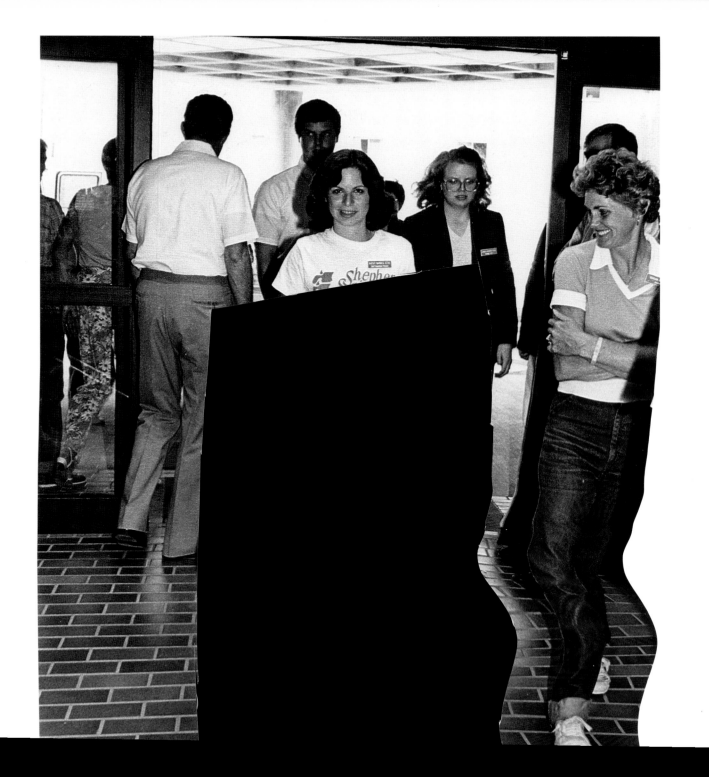

Pecans on Peachtree

The following announcement appeared in the November 1976 issue of *Courier Column*, the early predecessor of *Spinal Column*:

> THANKS ... to Marty Church, one of our faithful volunteers. Marty is selling shelled pecan halves for $3.00 per pound. The Buckhead Elks Auxiliary is sponsoring the sale with the proceeds being donated to Shepherd Spinal Center (SSC). Leave your order at the SSC desk and Marty will deliver the goodies on Thursday and Friday afternoons from now until December 15.

Such were the origins of one of the Shepherd Spinal Center Auxiliary's oldest and ~~~~fundraising traditions, Pecans on Peachtree. For five years, Marty Church would ~~~~~~handedly—to sell pecans for the benefit of Shepherd under the ~~~~~~~~~~~. But once the center was comfortably ensconced ~~~~~~~~~~~al holiday season pecan sale was taken over by ~~~~~y.

~~~~ Aftergut, one of Marty's early recruits and now ~~~~~y needed a fundraiser, and Pecans on Peachtree ~~~~~em at Peachtree Battle Shopping Center, just ~~~~~r she ran into." Cookie and the other early vol-~~~~~rs and hit the streets. "I'd take them to garden ~~~~~ce where there was a group of people."

~~~~ by marketing, and nobody has learned the les-~~~~al announcement (and order form) in *Spinal* ~~~~hotline, a toll-free number, and a website that ~~~~eral years, Cookie has done a television spot on ~~~~ successful pecan sales at the four Harris Teeter ~~~~t time, Pecans on Peachtree produced its own ~~~~course, anyone who drove anywhere near 2020 ~~~~er saw the huge hot-air balloon floating above ~~~~osolutely serious, "I'm gonna get on 'Oprah.'"

~~~~d Angel of the Year in 1995, Cookie has long ~~~~olunteers. Here's a story Cookie likes to tell, a ~~~~enter, and perhaps explains why people like ~~~~after the 1996 Paralympics she was asked to ~~~~ors ... who turned out to be female orthope-~~~~ng them through the Marcus Building—the ~~~~ center—when she noticed that one of them

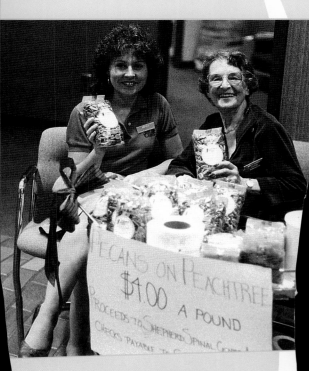

L-R: *Jane Bell and Marty Church.*

Also joining the staff was Dr. Robert Lathan as a staff internist with a special interest in respiratory problems. Dr. Lathan was instrumental in developing Shepherd's "No Smoking" policy, which made Shepherd Center smoke-free and contributed to a better environment for our patients—whom he encouraged to stop smoking.

⌒

Shepherd Spinal Center, intent on establishing itself as one of the premier spinal injury rehabilitation facilities in the country, wasted little time becoming fully operational. The new building offered opportunities for the kind of growth and expansion of services that had heretofore been merely the stuff of dreams.

By mid-summer, one of the new facility's most looked-for amenities was ready for use—the two-room dental suite, a gift of Mrs. Lindsey Hopkins, Jr. No longer would Shepherd patients with dental problems—or broken jaws—have to be transported to a dentist's office, with all the inconvenience and difficulty such an undertaking entailed. Not only could Shepherd patients now stay "home," but the special chair in the new suite was designed to facilitate transfer to and from a wheelchair. Under the direction of Dr. O. Anderson Currie, who had already been working with the center's patients for two years, the new suite made available most general dental procedures, along with such special services as mouth-stick fittings for quadriplegic patients.

Soon thereafter came the opening of the intensive care unit (ICU), officially inaugurated on November 15. This separate four-bed unit, immediately adjacent to the nursing station, was created for the special care of the center's most critical patients—acute spinal cord injuries, post-operative patients, patients on ventilators, and others requiring especially close observation. Equipped with the latest in patient monitoring technology, the new unit gave a boost to the center's effort to encourage earlier referral of spinal injury patients from all over the Southeastern region.

In fact, the opening of the ICU gave Shepherd's respiratory therapy program the opportunity to develop a specialty which continues to distinguish it to this day. According to Dr. James A. Settle, Shepherd's medical director of respiratory therapy, "We specialize in weaning patients off of ventilators whom other people have been unable to wean." Dr. Settle, a specialist in pulmonary medicine who began working at Shepherd in 1976, has gone on to build a department that includes two other doctors—Dr. Andrew Zadoff (now medical director of the intensive care unit) and Dr. David DeRuyter—one fulltime physician's assistant, and a contingent of therapists. "By now," says Dr. Settle today, "we have more experience with weaning than just about anybody, so we have patients referred to us from all over the country. Of course, critical care is part of our specialty, and most spinal cord centers don't take patients who are as acutely injured as some of our patients are, so we've had a unique opportunity to develop in this special area."

Early on we realized patients with compromised breathing capacity secondary to their spinal cord injury needed to be encouraged to quit smoking, which led to Shepherd Center becoming a smoke-free environment.

—Dr. Robert Lathan
Staff Internist

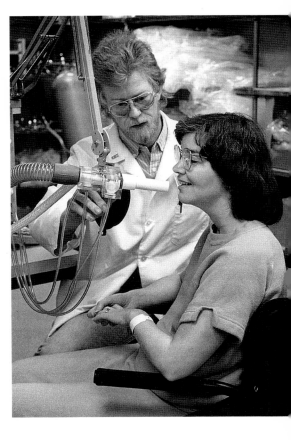

41

This most remarkable year in the life of Shepherd Spinal Center was not quite over yet. Also that fall, word came from the U.S. Department of Education's Rehabilitation Services Administration that Shepherd's application for $246,000 in grant funds had been approved. Of 50 facilities around the country submitting applications, only 17 were awarded grants. Furthermore, of the 17, Shepherd was one of just a couple, according to Dr. Apple, that achieved the distinction without the help of a university medical center affiliation. The significance of the award could hardly be overstated, especially since it meant official designation of Shepherd as one of the country's elite "model programs" in spinal injury rehabilitation. The grant afforded a "wonderful opportunity," continued Dr. Apple, "to make some great strides forward in areas previously left undeveloped through lack of funding."

The year officially came to a close with the naming of Tammy King, R.N., day charge nurse, as Shepherd Spinal Center's first Employee of the Year. One of the center's original employees (and currently the director of the new Marcus Community Bridge Program), Tammy was cited for her "untiring efforts under stress," her "outstanding example for the staff," and her "kindness, open-mindedness, and understanding." Given the events of 1982, merely having survived would seem grounds for exceptional commendation.

"Honey, how about dinner at Antoine's tonight?"
"Antoine's?"
"You know, in New Orleans."
"Well, sure. Why not?"
The dedication and creativity of Shepherd's volunteer community supplied some memorable highlights for 1983. Like, for instance, "Dinner at Antoine's," an affair to remember coordinated by the recently formed Special Projects Committee, headed by board members Danne Munford and Simon Selig. Eastern Airlines, taking the opportunity to showcase its new Boeing 757, sponsored the one-day round-trip excursion, while the sumptuous dinner with vintage wine was underwritten by Mr. and Mrs. Lindsey Hopkins, Jr. In another example of Shepherd's ripple effect, the person driving the project on Eastern's end, Regional Sales Manager Ken Stowe, was a close friend of John Shea, whose son David was a patient at Shepherd a year earlier.

Meanwhile, as the black-tie crowd boarded the Boeing, it was occurring to Mrs. Munford that there was a huge group of potential Shepherd Spinal Center supporters—specifically, the younger generation, James Shepherd's friends and all of their friends—for whom "Dinner at Antoine's" might not have exactly the right allure. Out of this thinking was born the Junior Committee, with inaugural chairmen Danny Yates and Betsy Akers, a group which over the years would prove enormously beneficial to the center's fundraising efforts.

The Juniors Step Up

According to Alana Shepherd, it was board member Danne Munford who in early 1983 first suggested that the "next generation" of Shepherd volunteers needed to get organized and get involved.

The Junior Committee, as it came to be called, was quick to respond. In May of that same year, and every May since then, the committee has put on its now-renowned Derby Day party, featuring food and drink, games and contests, huge-screen viewing of the Kentucky Derby, and, on into the evening, dancing to live music. Originally held at the Munfords' Rock Mill Farm in Alpharetta, then from 1988 to 1996 at Felix Cochran's Bluegrass development in Forsyth County, and for the last four years at Jim Richards' Foxhall Farm in Douglas County, the party now draws more than 5,500 revelers annually.

One of Shepherd's fundraising mainstays, Derby Day has now raised more than $2 million, and the event over the years has become the chief sponsor of the Wheelchair Division of the Peachtree Road Race. It also supports other therapeutic recreation programs like the annual Adventure Skills Workshop, a three-day camping trip to Alabama.

While the Junior Committee numbers well over two hundred active members each year, those who have served as chairmen of Derby Day should be mentioned —

1983: Betsy Akers and Danny Yates
1984: Sara Chapman and John Dryman
1985: Cathy Kupris Smith and John Dryman
1986: Anne Offen and Craig Jones
1987: Cathy Shepherd and Kevin Johnson
1988: Ann Teltsch and Tom Aderhold
1989: Elizabeth Smith and Steve Shepherd
1990: Lisa Carter DeGolian and Tommy Shepherd
1991: Elspeth Willcoxon and David Chalmers
1992: Donna Richardson and Spencer Smith, Jr.
1993: Lynn Grassell Nunnally and Talbot Nunnally
1994: Tricia McLean and Philip Millians
1995: Ansley Connor and Clay Willcoxon
1996: Ella Tyler and Steve Slade
1997: Lora Gray Fishman and Neil Conrad
1998: Molly Lanier and Gordon Bynum
1999: Pebbles Glenn and Malon Courts
2000: Mary Gilbreath and Dee King
2001: Elisabeth Estes and Ed Perry

Two new developments in 1983 reaffirmed Shepherd's dedication to treating more than the medical needs of its patients. Thanks to the generosity of the trustees of the Laura Shallenberger Trust, Jerry Gardner was named SSC's first chaplain. Acknowledging the critical importance of the spinal cord injured's spiritual needs, Jerry's duties included not only conducting weekly religious services, but also contacting each patient's own minister to ensure the best possible emotional and spiritual care.

Also this year, recognizing the truth that "it always helps to talk to someone who's been there," the peer support program began organizing under the leadership of Cindy Burns. A purely volunteer organization in its early days, peer support has grown to be one of the center's most visible programs. (See story, p. 133)

Nineteen eighty-three was also a year of much-deserved individual recognition, representing all three branches of SSC's organization. From the staff, Dr. David Apple was elected to serve a two-year term as the president of the American Spinal Injury Association (ASIA). With his election, Dr. Apple became the youngest person ever to preside over this organization of 275 spinal cord specialists from the United States and Canada. Representing the board of directors, Alana Shepherd received the Governors Award of "The Ones Who Care" Awards, sponsored by WXIA-TV. Cited for her service to the community through her years of work at SSC, Alana became the first woman to be so honored in the 10-year history of the awards. And, finally, from the ranks of the volunteers, Martha "Marty" Church, with over 4,000 hours of service to the hospital since its inception, was recognized as the Metropolitan Atlanta Volunteer of the Year by United Way. (See related story, p. 136)

But perhaps the year's most meaningful acknowledgment came to the hospital itself. Only 18 months after the new facility opened its doors—and several years earlier than anticipated—Shepherd Spinal Center was granted approval to expand into its shelled-in third floor to accommodate an additional 40 patient beds. The center's maxed-out occupancy, along with its ever-longer waiting list, constituted the ultimate accolade.

Raising the Roof

With the approval in hand, work on the third floor got underway immediately, and its completion—culminating in the dedication ceremony on May 23—was the big event for 1984.

The expansion was a tremendous step in Shepherd's growth—and its ability to provide the best and most thorough rehabilitation to its patients. A critical

al, " indicates that we are on the right track with our body of research."

Both inside and outside the hospital building, another program—less formal but no less integral to the life at Shepherd—continued to thrive in 1984. In May, renowned Atlanta artist John Feight and a corps of willing volunteers—including Shepherd patients, a men's exercise class from the Capital City Club, and Bank South employees—transformed the SSC-Piedmont tunnel into a passage through the jungle, complete with zebras, giraffes, parrots, butterflies, and jungle foliage. And outside, in the garden area along Peachtree Road, artist David Sampson's sculptured fountain was dedicated on October 17. Mr. Sampson, who was born with cerebral palsy and uses a wheelchair himself, designed this "Fountain of Life" in such a way that patients in wheelchairs could roll up to it and feel the water as it dripped off the sculpture.

The sculpture was commissioned by Mr. and Mrs. Lindsey Hopkins, Jr. in honor of their son, Lindsey Hopkins III, who served as president of the center during the construction of the new facility and who continues as a member of the advisory board. Indeed, many of the works of art throughout the hospital have come through the efforts of Lindsey III, who has generously supported Shepherd's efforts to ensure that art remains an essential part of the overall therapy program.

While still in the garden, though, and with Shepherd's commitment to total therapy in mind, it's a good time to note that also this month—October, 1984—Dotty Fuqua, advisory board member and former member of the board of directors, became the first recipient of the Shepherd Spinal Center Garden Therapy Award. The beautiful garden area along Peachtree Road, with its raised plant beds for patients involved in horticultural therapy, along with the original landscaping of the entire hospital grounds, were largely the result of Mrs. Fuqua's hard work as chairman of the Landscape Committee. Mr. and Mrs. Fuqua dedicated the landscaping at the front intrance in memory of their son Alan, who died in an airplane crash as a college student in 1971.

Not surprisingly, given the multitude of directions in which SSC was expanding, 1984 also saw the appointment of Jane Bell as the center's first director of volunteer services. With over 400 members of its volunteer corps, and more calling to get involved every day, the Auxiliary stepped forward to fund a full-time position which, it felt, had become a vital necessity.

Shepherd's Own Angels

While the concept of the Shepherd Angel made its first appearance in 1982, the idea took a few years to evolve into the very special expression of recognition that it represents today. In its earliest incarnation, the Angel took the form of holiday season ornaments and refrigerator magnets available for sale in the gift shop, but Shepherd's development office quickly saw the angel symbol as the perfect token of appreciation to volunteers and donors who had made special contributions for Shepherd's benefit.

"Then in 1985," says Alana Shepherd, "we had the idea of an Angel Luncheon, where we would officially gather to recognize the efforts of our special volunteers and contributors for the year, and at the same time we would pick one person as the Angel of the Year. That first year we chose Isobel Fraser, who had contributed toward the Isobel Fraser Wing for Patient Care on the third floor of the new Shepherd building."

To each year's honoree goes the beautiful Angel pin, elegant gold wings surrounding a diamond "S," commissioned by Maier & Berkele. The heavenly host of "Angels of the Year" includes:

1985: Isobel Fraser
1986: Virginia Crawford
1987: Reunette Harris
1988: Helen Lanier and Carol Lanier Goodman
1989: Billi Marcus
1990: Peggy Schwall
1991: Sara Chapman
1992: Anne DeBorde
1993: Claire Smith
1994: Jane Gibson
1995: Cookie Aftergut
1996: Marty Church and Paul Kennedy
1997: Edna Wardlaw
1998: Dottie Fuqua
1999: Sharon Umphenour
2000: Angie Marshall and Beverly Mitchell

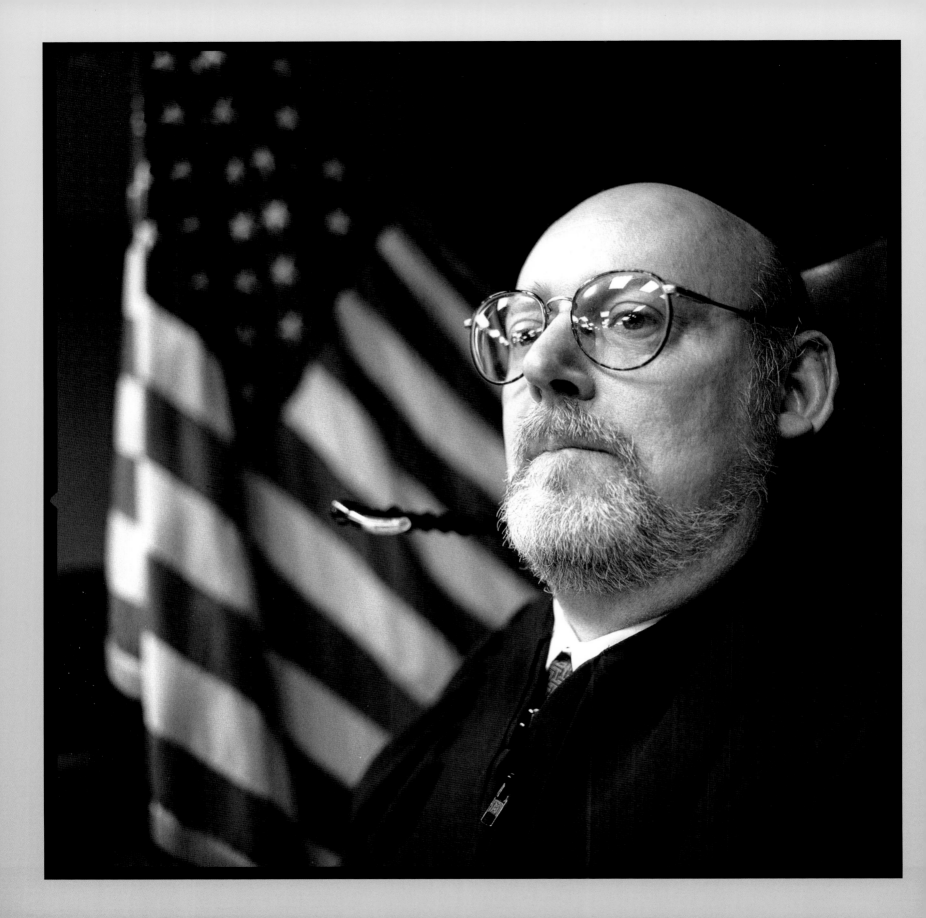

Charles Allen had everything going for him: a new job as an attorney with a Charleston, S.C., law firm, a lovely wife, two sons, and a new home. All that changed on November 12, 1982, when he fell off the back of a motorcycle going only five miles an hour. The freak accident broke his neck at the third cervical vertebra, leaving him quadriplegic.

Originally, Charles was dependent upon a ventilator to breathe, But Shepherd's Dr. Joseph Miller offered Charles the opportunity to be one of the first recipients of something called a phrenic pacer, a surgically implanted device that electrically stimulates the diaphragm muscles, helping paralyzed patients breathe.

"I have been off the ventilator since 1984," says Charles. "That operation was the factor that enabled me to lead a more active life."

His active life centers around his continued work in the legal profession—no longer as a lawyer but as a municipal court judge.

When he first considered returning to work, Charles asked several of his friends at the American Bar Association what kind of assistance the ABA offered to attorneys with disabilities. The answer was that the ABA had no policies concerning lawyers with disabilities, so Charles's friends formed the Handicapped Lawyers Committee. Thanks to the committee's work, the ABA now offers a clearinghouse of information to attorneys with disabilities throughout the United States and also serves as a powerful advocate for the rights of members of the bar with disabilities.

But as for himself, says Charles today, "I am more inclined to encourage people to become active. I have not been an advocate as such, in the sense of going to court and seeking rights for people with disabilities. I seem to prefer to invest my time and emotions in the people themselves, encouraging them to achieve, rather than lobbying the government."

Charles's personal life has also been rewarding. After being divorced for more than a decade, he married Jean Keil in October 1998. His two sons are now grown. The older, Lee, graduated from the University of South Carolina and now works in Idaho, where he leads young people with substance abuse problems on Outward Bound-type recovery adventures. Matthew is studying culinary arts at Johnson & Wales University, and, more important, has produced the family's first grandchild, Kye. The delighted grandfather admits that Kye "is the object of a lot of attention these days."

His time at Shepherd, Charles says, "was in retrospect essential, in terms of providing the process of acknowledging my situation and developing strategies for adapting to it. The expertise and quality of care at Shepherd permitted me to look inward to begin the long process of coming to terms with my disability. I don't know any other place that would have afforded me such a safe and secure environment to make that huge adjustment."

Today Charles says he has much to be thankful for. "I have been remarkably well physically, and that is a wonderful blessing. And I am deeply grateful for the time I've had to watch my sons grow up. In fact, I have said many times that I would rather be where I am right now than where I was before my accident. I have been blessed in many ways."

(Thanks to Dianne Witter's profile, "Charles Allen: Surpassing the Odds," Spinal Column, Winter 1990, pp. 13-14)

Charles Allen

"I have said many times that I would rather be where I am right now than where I was before my accident. I have been blessed in many ways."

Ten Years Young . . .

SC's tenth year got off to a typically breathtaking start with the announcement of a $500,000 gift from Virginia C. Crawford, money which would make possible what was hailed as "the crowning achievement of the expansion program"—the Virginia Carroll Crawford Nutrition Centers.

The new cafeteria and serving grills on each patient floor constituted nothing less than a revolution in hospital food service: freedom of choice, on-the-spot selection of foods, meals cooked to order, second helpings—amenities all the more desirable in that spinal cord injured patients tend to lose weight after their injuries and need encouragement to put those pounds back on. No wonder patients at the February 13 dedication celebration wore "I Love Virginia" t-shirts and waved heart-shaped signs reading "No More Hospital Trays!" and "Eggs Cooked to Order!"

This tenth anniversary year also witnessed another memorable dedication ceremony—that of the Cecil B. Day, Sr. Memorial Greenhouse, the generous gift of Mrs. Deen Day Smith. This fully accessible structure, large enough to accommodate up to a half dozen wheelchairs, gave yet another boost to SSC's thriving horticultural therapy program. With its work tables high enough for wheelchairs to roll under and climate-controlled environment, the greenhouse would mean year-round classes for gardening-minded patients.

When a research study of 200 former patients revealed that 71 percent had been employed before their injury and only 17 percent were employed up to five years after discharge, yet another component of total rehabilitation was brought clearly into focus. Not surprisingly, vocational services, as it is now called, has evolved into one of Shepherd's most innovative and successful programs. (See story, p. 96.)

In fact, 1985 was a promising year for a number of programs emerging from the ongoing work of the research department:

The outdoor program, begun in 1984 under the direction of George Holland, was created in direct response to a research department survey of discharged patients indicating a prevalent desire to become more involved is such physical activities as hunting, fishing, water sports, and camping. Entering its second

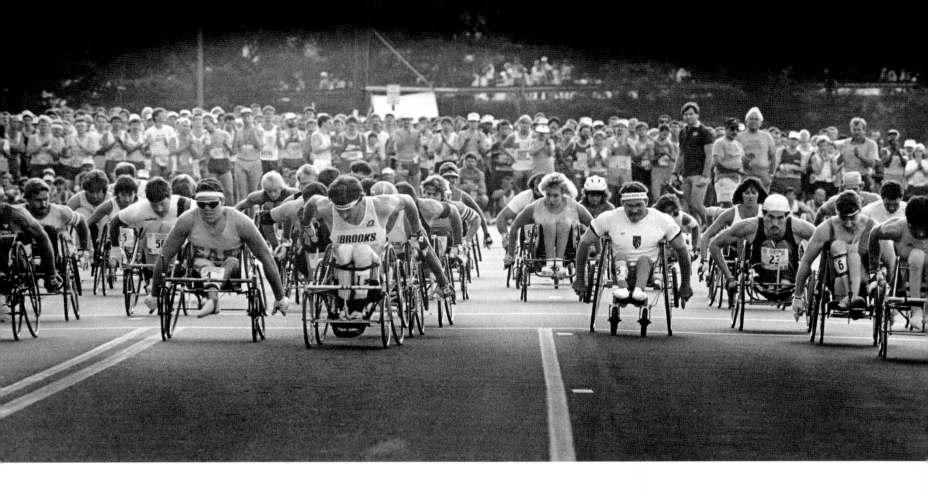

race competition held at venues around the nation.

The Wheelchair Division had become a distinct component of the Peachtree Road Race in 1982, and Shepherd had been increasingly involved in coordinating and promoting the race since 1983. But for the 1986 race, Shepherd received "official" sponsorship status, giving the center responsibility for sending invitations to the athletes, arranging their travel, ground transportation, and hotel accommodations, hosting a post-race brunch, and, of course, awarding prize money for the top finishers. Shepherd—with some support from Invacare—would also foot the bill, thanks in large part to the efforts of the SSC Auxiliary.

Typical of Shepherd's innovative and far-reaching approach to serving the disabled community, its enthusiastic sponsorship of the Wheelchair Division of the PRR would prove to be important preparation for a much greater effort to be undertaken a decade later.

At about the same time the racers were wheeling to the starting line, Shepherd was piloting yet another new program: SPARX (Shepherd's Program About Real X-periences), a part of the spina bifida program. Originally, the 120-

Like Alana, James is a tremendous visionary. He's always looking way down the road, and that's what drives Shepherd. There are always new ideas, and the momentum never slows. We always feel like we can do it better.

—Sara Chapman
Member, Board of Directors

hour summer program was targeted to self-motivated young people with spina bifida between the ages of 10 and 20, giving them the opportunity to learn new recreation skills, develop new friendships, and increase their independence. Like so many successful Shepherd programs, SPARX has grown, evolved, and customized itself to the needs of the children and adolescents it serves. By the time it celebrated its tenth anniversary, SPARX was offering a range of summer sessions, lasting from one to three weeks each, for five different age-specific groups.

Four years and one month after the grand opening on Peachtree Road, the entrance to Shepherd Spinal Center received a finishing touch. On that date, May 22, 1986, Terry Lee, with the tug of a rope, unveiled the larger-than-life bronze image of himself that has become SSC's sculptural—and inspirational—centerpiece.

Commissioned by an anonymous donor and created by renowned sculptor Ed Dwight, the statue—depicting Lee hurling a javelin—stands impressively at the Shepherd building's portico entrance, commanding attention and at the same time offering silent encouragement to anyone entering the hospital.

And no wonder. Despite being paralyzed in a hunting accident when he was 13, Terry has led a life of remarkable achievement by any standard. In addition to his successful career with Adams/Cates Realty, he has competed internationally in wheelchair athletic events and earned the gold medal as the Pentathlon champion in the 1983 National Wheelchair Games in Hawaii. Adding even more depth to this rich and eventful life has been Terry's tireless work with the Youth Wheelchair Sports Program in DeKalb, Gwinnett, and Cobb counties. The enthusiasm of these youngsters, says Terry, "is marvelous to see."

Meanwhile, two important gifts were announced from Shepherd's network of devoted benefactors. Mrs. Elizabeth H. Irby, in memory of her husband Alton F. Irby, and Mrs. Reunette W. Harris, in the name of herself and her late husband W. Clair Harris, both contributed substantially to the vital Patient Equipment Endowment Fund. The purpose of the fund is the purchase of basic and state-of-the-art adaptive equipment—often quite costly—for the many patients who lack the financial resources themselves. These two generous gifts gave a tremendous boost to the center's announced goal of $2.5 million to fully endow the fund.

In fact, as 1986 came to a close, Mrs. Harris was paid special honor by the board of directors, both for her contribution to the Patient Equipment Endowment Fund as well as her generous donation to what would thenceforth be known as the Reunette W. and W. Clair Harris Patient Wing. Located on the Shepherd Building's third floor, the wing includes 16 fully accessible patient rooms along with four of the center's eight intensive care unit beds.

The following year, 1987, saw the first-ever publication of SSC's annual report.

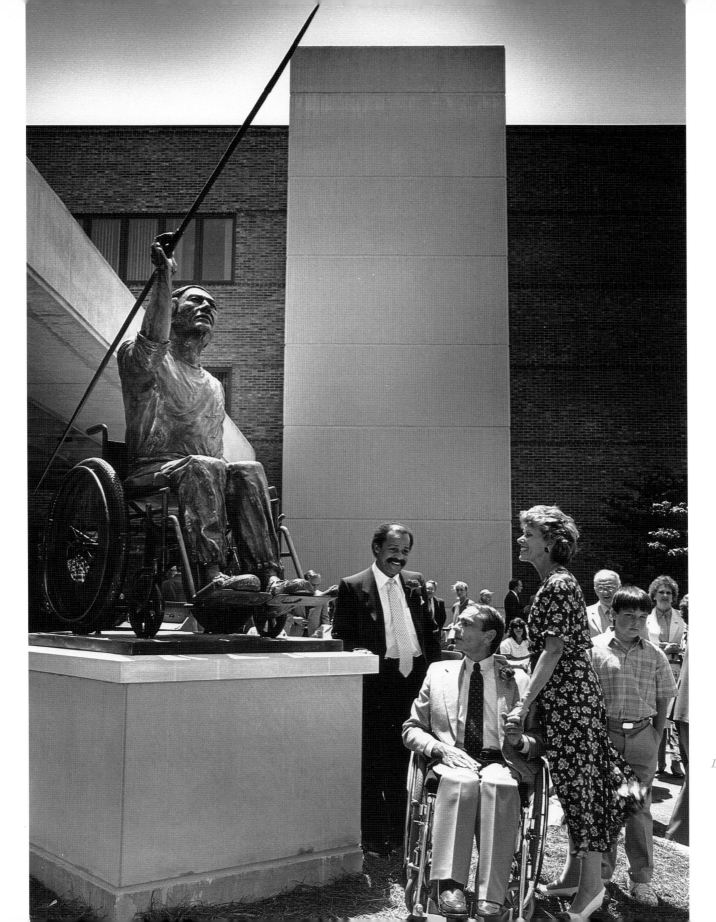

L-R: Ed Dwight (sculptor), Terry Lee, and Alana Shepherd.

55

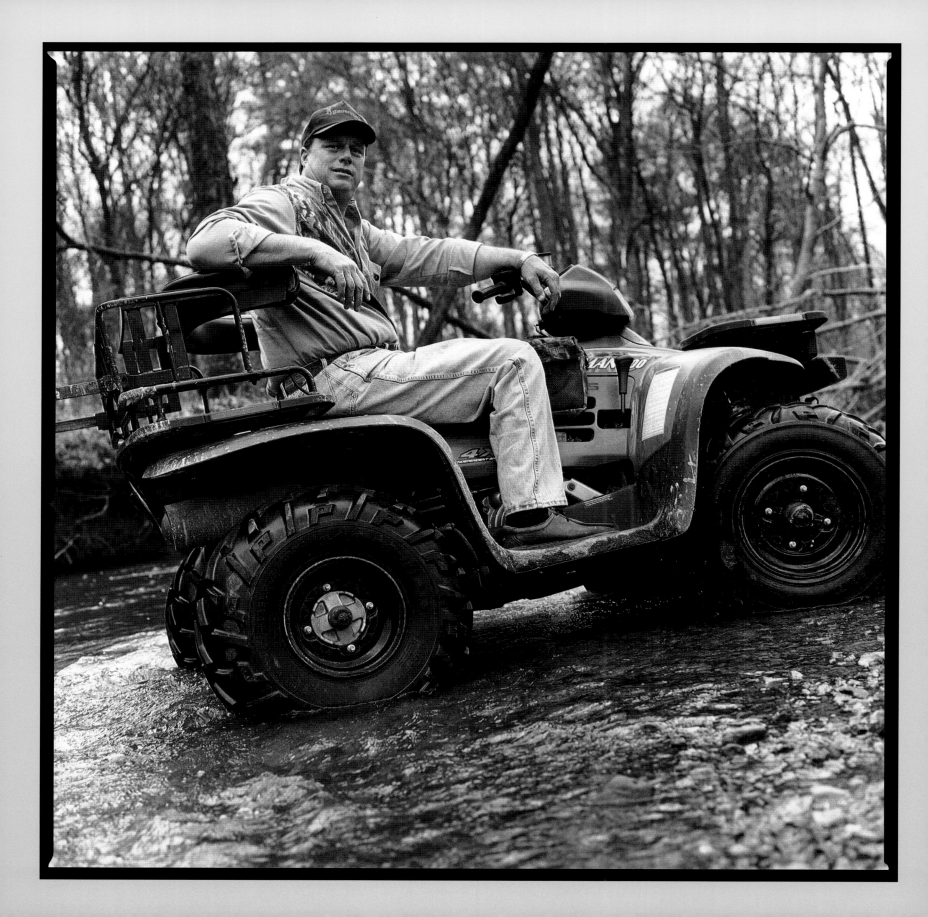

"I fell asleep on my deer stand," says David Renz, recalling the 1985 accident that left him paraplegic. "When I woke up, I was on the ground. I had fallen head-first onto my gun." The gun broke, but David was able to fire it three times to signal for help. "I was in excruciating pain. I couldn't breathe or move. I remember thinking I might die. I was 30 years old, I had a brand new baby girl less than a month old, and a wonderful wife who'd been my high school sweetheart. I didn't want to die."

After brief stays in two hospitals, David was transferred to Shepherd, where he successfully went through the vigorous rehab program that allowed him to return to his very busy life in Dalton, Georgia.

"Well, Rocky Face, actually," says David today, describing the town as "a big metropolis between Dalton and Tunnel Hill." He and his family live on 20 acres there — "my own wildlife plantation," he calls it — where he does all the plowing, mowing, "and everything else." David bought the land seven years ago and finished building his house four years ago.

"We planned the house for about ten years," he says, "and it's just what we wanted. A single-story ranch, fully accessible. I designed it myself, drew the whole thing on a piece of paper."

As for the one-month old-daughter, she's now a freshman in high school, and David recently enjoyed the keen parental pleasure of escorting her to her place of honor on the Homecoming Court.

Though his farm is five miles away, David's busy professional and community life is still centered in Dalton. Since his injury, David has served as a youth leader and deacon at Dalton's First Presbyterian Church; he has been area chairman for Ducks Unlimited, a wetlands fundraising organization; he's been a board member and treasurer for the Creative Arts Guild; and he's been deeply involved in the Dalton/Whitfield Disability Awareness Council.

Currently, says David, "I was just put on the board of directors of United Way, where I'm the funds distribution chairman. I'm also membership chairman for our local Kiwanis Club. And probably the most time-consuming of my present activities is being chairman of the new state-wide Brain and Spinal Injury Trust Fund that the governor just set up. I'm putting a whole lot of time into that." (In 1998 the Georgia Legislature raised drunk driving fines by 10 percent and directed that monies raised by the surcharge be channeled into the Trust Fund, to be applied to the long-term costs associated with brain and spinal cord injuries.)

If there's a downside, says David, "I'm not doing as much hunting as I'd like to do. Maybe I can get out more this year."

David also admits to not being as involved in Shepherd's Junior Committee as he used to be. "I'm getting too old to be a "junior" anymore," he says.

But make no mistake. David Renz is not slowing down.

(Thanks to Sarah Hicks' profile of David, "Making Life Meaningful," Spinal Column, Winter 1996, pp. 22-23)

David Renz

"I was 30 years old, I had a brand new baby girl less than a month old, and a wonderful wife who'd been my high school sweetheart. I didn't want to die."

This document, a five-page special supplement in the fall issue of *Spinal Column*, came roughly at the midpoint of the center's 25-year history and underscored with bold strokes the phenomenal growth and achievements of the institution. A few highlights from the report of fiscal year April 1, 1986—March 31, 1987:

- Shepherd was the nation's largest facility specializing exclusively in spinal cord disorders.
- Shepherd was one of only 13 hospitals nationally that are federally designated as "models of care" for others to follow.
- For the fiscal year, inpatient admissions totaled 418 (compared to 236 just two years earlier.
- Outpatients numbered 4,272 for the year (compared to 2,850 two years earlier).
- Average occupancy rate for the 80-bed hospital stood at 88 percent.
- The center served patients from 20 states (stretching from Florida to Alaska), as well as from Belgium, Brazil, and Canada.

In accounting for the underlying causes for Shepherd's remarkable success, however, perhaps the most telling statistic was the hospital's staffing ratio. While the ratio of patients to staff in a general, non-specialized hospital setting was approximately three to one, the ratio at Shepherd stood at four staff members to each patient.

In his introduction to the report, Jim Collins, hired as SSC's first salaried administrator during the move to Peachtree Road, summed it up nicely: "Our quest for excellence is no longer a dream; it is a reality."

The annual report also revealed another interesting statistic, one which bore directly upon the center's increasing effort in the area of injury prevention. Of all in-patient admissions during the fiscal year, 37 percent were the result of automobile accidents, and of those injured, fewer than 1 percent were buckled up at the time of the accident. Following up the injury prevention program's production of "The Time It Takes," Dr. David Apple in 1987 became honorary chairman and spokesman for the Georgia Safety Belt Coalition, whose overriding purpose was to get a mandatory seatbelt law enacted by the Georgia legislature.

Speaking to the *Atlanta Constitution's* Bill Shipp, whom he enlisted in the cause, Dr. Apple put the case succinctly: "I see scores of serious spinal injuries each year, almost 40 percent of which result from auto accidents. By simply using safety belts, a person can cut the chances of death or serious injury in half."

Unhappily, while the bill introduced in the 1987 session by Senators Paul Coverdell and Culver Kidd sailed through the Senate, the legislation was defeated by the House Motor Vehicles Committee, the members of which appeared unwilling to intrude upon the "personal rights" of Georgia's citizens. Dr. Apple

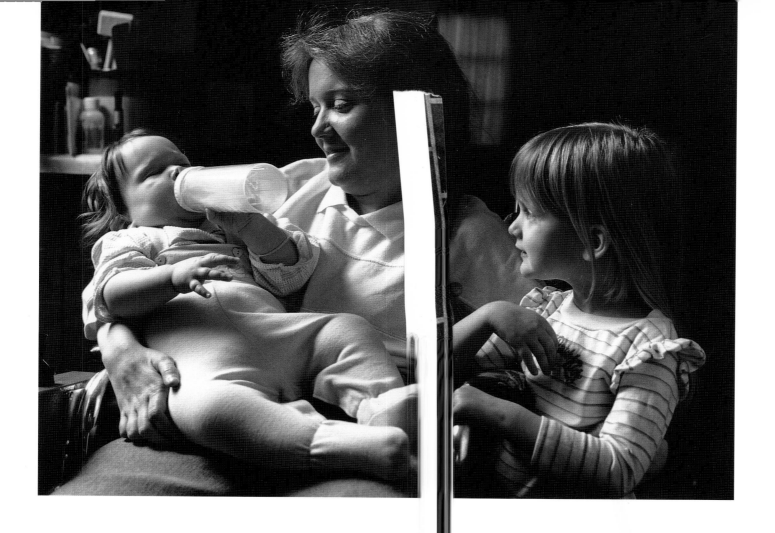

vowed to return to the state house door, however, and the legis   e did in fact enact a seatbelt law in 1988.

On the medical front, Dr. Bruce Green announced the inc   n of a fertility program at Shepherd, dramatically improving the once-dis   rognosis for fertility in spinal cord injured males. Dr. Green, the center's m   l director of urology, credited the pioneering work of the University of Mic   's Dr. Carol Bennett, who, as a visiting professor at SSC, shared her EES (el   timulation) technology with Dr. Green and his staff.

Meanwhile, from the development office came word of the   ointment of Dell Sikes as Shepherd's new director of development. Forme   fundraising executive at Georgia Tech, Dell joined Shepherd on November   t in time to begin spreading the word that . . . "The Best Is Yet to Come."

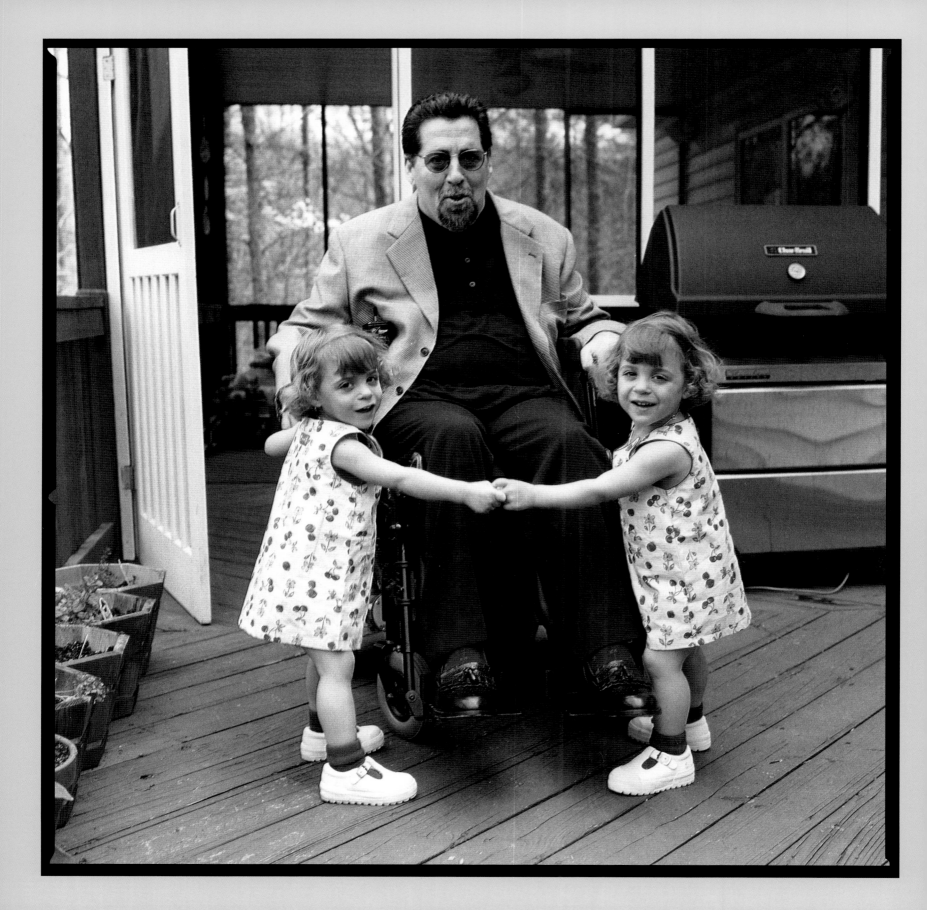

*T*hirteen years ago, Atlanta police detective James J. ("J. J.") Biello walked into his own nightmare. Trying to thwart a robbery at a restaurant in Buckhead, he was gunned down at close range. One of the assailant's bullets sliced through his vocal cords to the fourth cervical vertebra in his spinal cord, leaving him quadriplegic.

As is usually the case when a police office is injured in the line of duty, the community rallied to offer support. J.J. and Richard Williams, another officer shot at about the same time, were hailed at "Friends of Biello and Williams," a fundraising celebration at Piedmont Park, and both officers were recognized by then-Governor Joe Frank Harris.

But all the community support in the world wasn't going to undo the damage that had been inflicted upon this active, athletic police officer. For J.J., the future suddenly looked very different, and not very inviting. "Trust me," he says today. "It was difficult — for me, for my family. Your whole life has been shattered."

J.J. wasn't about to quit, though, and in 1990, three years after his injury, his new career was established with his election to the Cherokee County Commission. He had campaigned vigorously for 10 months, a task made all the more difficult by his limited mobility. "I couldn't hold the microphone," he said after that first victory, "but I had better ideas, and that was the point I wanted to make." The voters responded, giving him 54 percent of the vote in the primary and an overwhelming 68 percent in the general election.

"I worked hard," said J.J., "to let the constituency know that, although I've had a dramatic change in my lifestyle, I'm not a quitter."

Ten years later, they're still getting the message. In the year 2000, J.J. was elected to his fourth consecutive term as commissioner, so he'll be serving the good people of Cherokee County at least until the end of 2003.

"I'm happy in the commissioner's office," J.J. says today, "but I'm not going to say that I don't have any further political ambitions. In fact, right now I'm working hard to be appointed by Governor Barnes to the state boxing commission. I've loved the sport for years."

There's also a full plate of community work. J.J. served as chairman of the building committee of St. Michael's Church in Woodstock, and, apart from his government job, he's also the chairman of the Cherokee County Recreation Authority.

In the meantime, J.J. has become a grandfather. His older son, who works for IBM, is the father of twin two-year-old girls. His younger son, still unmarried, works as a karate instructor.

J.J. looks back at his time at Shepherd as an "extremely difficult six months. At the injury level I had, there wasn't but so much they could do for me." But he came through those difficult days with plenty of determination: "I wasn't going to let anybody just take everything from me. The guy who shot me down wasn't going to take everything."

And in the rebuilding of his life, he learned two lessons well worth passing along: "First, the big secret to handling an injury like this is to stay busy. And second, for me, it was very important to go mainstream. I really wanted to be out there — especially for young people. Young people who are injured need to understand that you can still live, that there is still something you can do."

(Thanks to Lisa M. Cape's profile of J. J. Biello in "Public Service Takes a New Twist," Spinal Column, Spring 1991, pp. 6-7.)

J. J. Biello

"Young people who are injured need to understand that you can still live, that there is still something you can do."

The Best is Yet to Come

*W*hen 12-year-old Megan Apple, Dr. Apple's daughter, released a thousand orange, white, and green balloons into the air on May 3, 1988, the past converged with the future. Megan was one week old when her father helped open the doors of Shepherd Spinal Center in 1975. And this day in May marked a new beginning: ground-breaking for the $23 million, 153,000-square-foot expansion that would more than double the center's size and cement its reputation as the nation's largest hospital specializing in spinal disorders.

Key components of the expansion—which began with the construction of a badly needed parking deck at the rear of the property—were the addition of 20 inpatient beds, a much-enlarged outpatient department, and a world-class therapeutic recreation complex that would include an indoor swimming pool, a full-size gymnasium, a weight room, an elevated indoor track over the gym, and a comprehensive arts and crafts area.

If such plans seemed ambitious—or even extravagant—the expansion was simply a manifestation of the Shepherd vision, and a resounding reaffirmation of its mission to restore spinal injured patients to full participation in the world from which they had been temporarily displaced. As Alana told the *Northside Neighbor*, "We must continue to strengthen the services supporting our patients' often fragile transition from being a patient to being a vital member of the community. And, in turn, as we send more and more patients back to their homes, we must be able and ready to support them with superior outpatient services. Our goal for the new building is really a promise to the patients that we are committed to serve and that the best is yet to come."

The Home Depot chairman and SSC board member Bernard "Bernie" Marcus was selected to head the Expansion Campaign Committee, which, raising as its banner "The Best Is Yet to Come," announced a $12 million fundraising goal.

Never reluctant to aim for such goals, the Shepherd community of friends and volunteers enlisted in the campaign with their accustomed enthusiasm. By the time the Junior Committee's Derby Day (chaired by Ann Teltsch and Tom Aderhold and held for the first time at Felix Cochran's Bluegrass development in Forsyth County)

Somebody asked me, "Doesn't it bother you trying to raise $12 million?" I said, no, it doesn't bother me at all. I'm gonna let Alana and the Lord worry about that. And in two years they had done it.

—Harold Shepherd
Founding Board Member

Opposite, L-R:
Fred Alias, James Shepherd,
Bernie Marcus, and Henry
Smith (Architect)

62

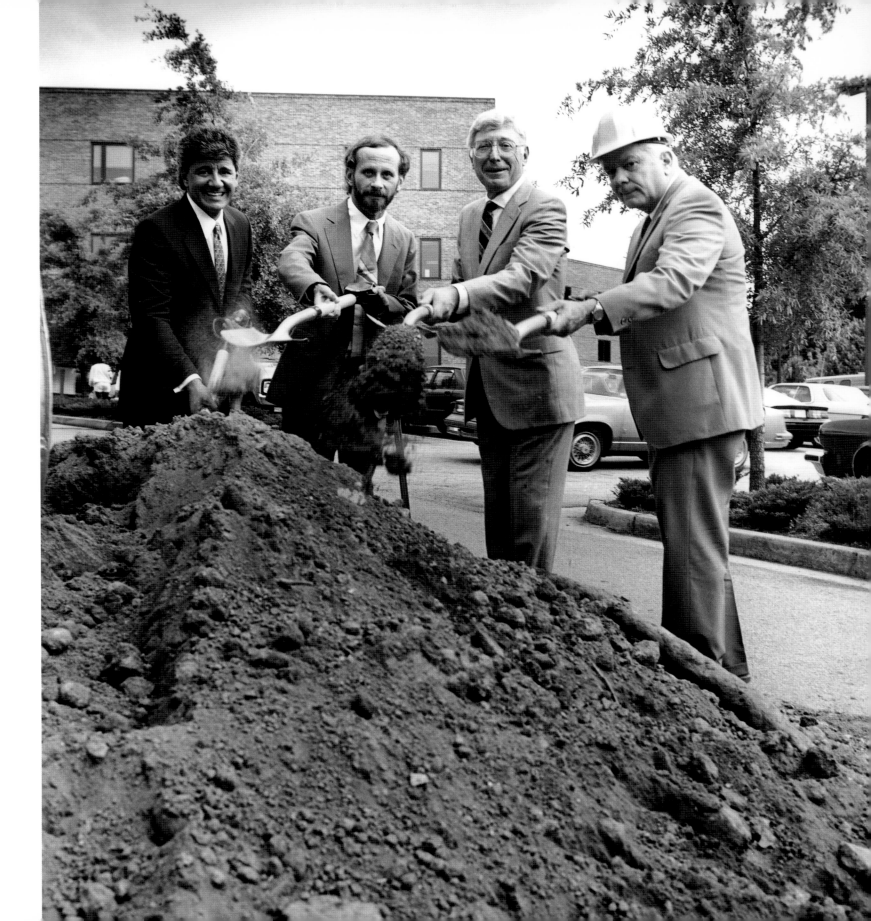

made its $100,000-plus contribution, donations had already exceeded the $4 million mark. Meanwhile, RTM, the largest franchisee of Arby's Roast Beef Restaurants, offered itself as the title sponsor of the annual golf tournament, and in the absence of John and Shirley Shea, who had been the driving force behind the tournament for three years, Billi Marcus and Jim Groome stepped up to the tee box. The new formula worked: The RTM Challenge contributed another $120,000 to the campaign.

New ground was being broken inside the hospital as well. With less fanfare, perhaps, than the outdoor event, but every bit as integral to SSC's mission, Mark Johnson was hired as the center's advocacy coordinator. Actually created as a part-time position in October 1987, Mark's advocacy office focuses on issues that affect the entire disabled community—accessibility, in particular—and underscores Shepherd's commitment to the quality of life of people with disabilities, a commitment that endures long after patients leave the hospital.

For example, with the blessing of SSC, which realized the importance of the issues being raised, Mark played a pivotal role in coordinating the effort to make the 1988 Democratic National Convention, held in Atlanta, accessible to the 87 conventioneers who needed assistance. Working with the City of Atlanta Task Force on Disabled Persons, Mark's corps of more than one hundred volunteers effected such permanent changes in the local landscape as additional curb cuts at the Omni/World Congress Center, increased accessibility of the CNN Center, and improved training of Metropolitan Atlanta Rapid Transit Authority (MARTA) drivers who operate the lift-equipped buses for people in wheelchairs. But in his fight for a barrier-free Atlanta—and for disability rights nationwide— Mark Johnson was just getting started. (See story, p. 74.)

Overcoming barriers, of course, is SSC's ongoing narrative, and two members of the Shepherd community added fascinating chapters to the story in 1988. Founding board member Clark Harrison, who in 1985 had successfully flown solo to Alaska and back—and in the process raised more than $12,000 for the center, decided this year to help raise money for the expansion by piloting his Cherokee 140, "The Spirit of Shepherd," to Stolberg, Germany, where he had been paralyzed by a sniper's bullet in World War II. The goodwill mission came to an unexpected end when difficult weather blew Clark off-course and forced him to crash-land on the rocky coast of Greenland, but Clark somehow survived the crash virtually unscathed.

The other story of the year was that of Bill Furbish, a C-7 quadriplegic as a result of a dive into the Ogeechee River in 1985, the week of his graduation from Georgia Southern University. Having always been an outstanding athlete, Bill became interested in wheelchair athletics during his rehabilitation. Shepherd's therapeutic recreation department fueled his interest by providing information on wheelchair racing and loaning him his first racing chair, and in November 1986 he won his first championship.

The RTM Challenge

In June 1984 the Majik Market Celebrity Golf Tournament raised $12,700 to "Raise the Roof" at Shepherd; that is, to help the center expand into the third floor of its still relatively new building on Peachtree Road.

Two key volunteers in that effort, John and Shirley Shea, knew a good thing when they saw it. The following year, without Majik Market's affiliation, they worked with John Gerring, golf pro at Atlanta Country Club, to organize a "second annual golf tournament for Shepherd," which raised $30,000 for the center. Over the next two years, still under John and Shirley's direction, the annual golf tournament raised another $200,000 for Shepherd. And yet another remarkably successful fundraising tradition was firmly established.

In 1988, with the Sheas' decision to turn their volunteer efforts elsewhere, the golf tournament got a new sponsor and a new name—The RTM Challenge—and new chairmen, Billi Marcus and Jim Groome. It was Billi who suggested the sponsorship to RTM senior vice president Dennis Cooper, who happened to be her neighbor; he signed on for three years, but the arrangement has lasted for 13—and counting.

RTM ("Results Through Motivation"), the largest franchisee of Arby's Roast Beef restaurants and the owner of Mrs. Winner's Fried Chicken restaurants, has helped make the annual golf tournament a huge success—offering not only financial support but also planning, design and printing services, and gifts for players. Dennis Cooper and John Gray, VP for marketing and communications, have given their time and enthusiasm to the event in every one of the 13 tournaments.

While the site of The RTM Challenge has been variable (the Atlanta Country Club, Atlanta Athletic Club, the Golf Club of Georgia, Cherokee Country Club, and, for the last four years, Chateau Elan have all hosted the event), the leadership of Billi Marcus and Julian Mohr (co-chairmen since 1991) has remained constant. Thanks to their tireless devotion, The RTM Challenge has contributed close to $2.5 million dollars to Shepherd Center.

In its first years, monies raised by the tournament were earmarked for the expansion project, which would upon its completion be named The Billi Marcus Building, at least in part as a tribute to her unstinting volunteer work, which began in earnest in 1987. Subsequent beneficiaries of the RTM event have been the Patient Outreach Fund and vocational services.

Tournament Planning Committee

Billi Marcus
Co-Chair

Julian Mohr
Co-Chair

Joe Chapman
Dennis Cooper
John Gray
Audrey Greenwood
Jim Groome
Becky Hall
Carol Sue Legum
Janice Mathia
Linda Meltz
Rick O'Callaghan
Caryl Paller
Jeanne Privette
Frank Spears
Clay Willcoxon
Judy Zaban

65

By 1988, now back at Shepherd working as an assistant data processing manager, Bill had won 30 gold medals in U.S. competition and had set five national records. This stellar success led to more remarkable achievement. He was selected as one of 145 American athletes to be on the U.S. Disabled Sports Team participating in the 1988 Paralympics, and in October Bill returned from the games in Seoul, Korea, with a gold medal in the 100-meter relay and a bronze in the 100-meter race.

With the $23 million expansion on the front burner, the fundraising campaign occupied premium space in SSC's collective consciousness throughout 1989. News from the development office was encouraging. By late spring, private contributions had reached the $9 million mark, well on the way to the $12 million goal. Dell Sikes announced at the same time a $500,000 challenge grant from an anonymous donor, payable when the goal was reached.

Before the year was out, he would announce yet another half-million-dollar pledge, a gift from the Livingston Foundation, the private family foundation begun by Roy and Bess Livingston. The Livingstons, whose daughter Lesley Livingston Keller had been a college classmate of Alana Shepherd and advisory board chairman Peggy Schwall, were among the first and most generous supporters of SSC. In recognition of their tremendous contribution, the gymnasium in the new building would be named the Livingston Gymnasium.

Meanwhile, on the volunteer front, hospital lore has it that in early 1989 a world-weary member of the Special Projects Committee said, "Can't I just write a big check without having to fly off somewhere?" Thus was born the Legendary Party, which, after months of planning, was inaugurated on November 18 at the Westin Lenox Hotel. Under the magical direction of chairman Sally Tomlinson—and to the delight of armchair travelers—Italy came to Atlanta for the evening, in the form of a Venetian masquerade ball. By all accounts the first annual Legendary Party lived up to its billing—and would continue to do so. (See accompanying story)

Also this year, the three volunteer fundraising mainstays—the Auxiliary, led by President Ann Carter McDonald (wife of Dr. Allen McDonald); the Junior Committee, chaired by Elizabeth Smith and Steve Shepherd; and The RTM Challenge, again directed by Billi Marcus and Jim Groome—each contributed in excess of $100,000, with virtually all of the monies earmarked for the new expansion.

In another story from outside the center's walls, 1989 brought heightened prestige to the Shepherd Spinal Center Wheelchair Division of the Peachtree Road Race. For the first time, the race was named the National 10K Championship Road Race by the National Wheelchair Athletic Association—meaning that when Craig Blanchette and Sharon Hedrick (winners of the men's and women's open divisions) rolled across the finish line, they earned the title "National Champion" in their race category.

A Legend in It's Own Time

Immediately upon its inception in November 1989, the Legendary Party became a highlight of Atlanta's fall social season.

Thanks to the Shepherd Auxiliary, and to the tireless efforts of innumerable volunteers, the Legendary Party has raised close to $4 million for such special Shepherd programs as the Patient Care Endowment Fund, the Patient Equipment Fund, assistive technology, MS research, the acquired brain injury program, and building renovations and additions.

A nod of appreciation to those who have played a prominent role in the success of the Legendary Party —

1989—"Ballo Veneziano"
   Sally Tomlinson, Chairman
   Virginia Crawford, Honorary Chairman
1990—"A Medieval Affair"
   Sissy Wright, Chairman
   Helen S. Lanier, Honorary Chairman
1991—"Camelot"
   Sharon Umphenour, Chairman
   Billi and Bernie Marcus, Honorary Chairmen
1992—"Cinderella's Ball"
   Peggy Schwall and Claire Smith, Chairmen
   Deen Day and Charles Smith, Honorary Chairmen
1993—"The Legend of 1,001 Nights"
   Becky Robinson Smith, Chairman
   Marsha and Martin Marchman, Co-Chairmen
   Alana Shepherd, Honorary Chairman
1994—"Song of the Muses"
   Elizabeth Allen, Chairman; Lois Puckett, Co-Chairman
   Peggy and Emory Schwall, Honorary Chairmen
1995—"Evening on the Nile"
   Vicki Scaljon, Chairman; Claire Smith, Co-Chairman
   Jane and Dr. David Apple, Honorary Chairmen
1996—"A Secret Garden"
   Beverly Mitchell, Chairman; June Hunter, Co-Chairman
   Alice Richards, Honorary Chairman
1997—"Phantoms of Venice"
   Joy Stuart, Chairman; Jane Apple, Co-Chairman
   William C. Fowler, Honorary Chairman
1998—"The Legend of the Celts" (10th year)
   The previous nine chairmen listed above served as co-chairs
   James Shepherd, Honorary Chairman
1999—"Legend of the Firebird"
   Anne Hux, Chair; Ruth Dobbs Anthony, Chair-Elect
   Emmy and Carl Knobloch, Honorary Chairmen
2000—"Spirit of Paris"
   Ruth Dobbs Anthony, Chair; Valery Voyles Singleton, Chair-Elect
   Ruth Dobbs McDonald, Honorary Chair

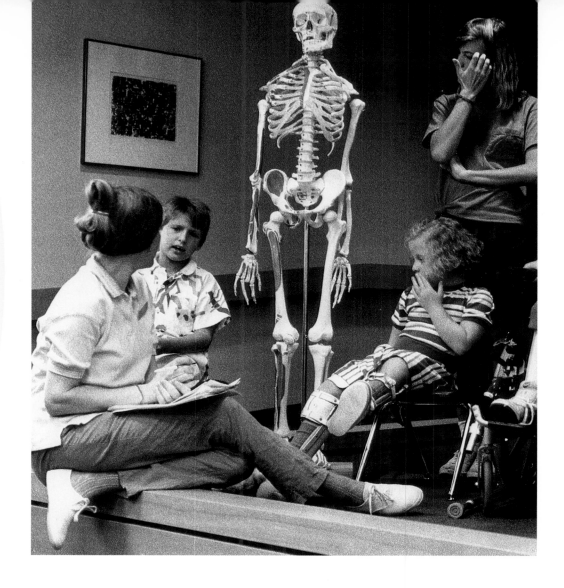

Before the year was out, Shepherd was piloting yet another program and again expanding its mission to restore the spinal injured to full and independent life: the transitional living program for young adults with spina bifida. The new program targeted the significant number of people with spina bifida reaching young adulthood who were mentally and physically able to live on their own, but who had been dependent upon their parents their whole lives and hadn't developed the basic skills necessary for independent living.

The crucial first step toward independence would be a transitional living phase, where these adults would have "a highly structured environment in which to 'practice' independence." The ultimate goal of the program, beyond independence, is the gainful employment that makes an individual a true member of the community. "We help them explore their vocational interests," explained Judy

In Memorium:
Clark Harrison
(d. March 28, 1989)

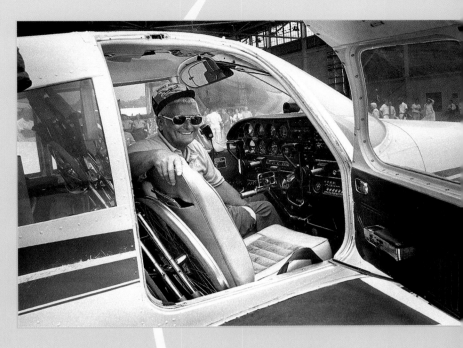

Founding board member Clark Harrison was felled by a sniper's bullet in Germany during WWII, but though the injury left him paralyzed below the waist, it did not impede a life of remarkable achievement.

A lifelong Decatur resident, Clark served as a DeKalb County commissioner from 1956 to 1960 and as commission chairman from 1969 to 1972. He was chairman of Fidelity National Bank and was a driving force behind bringing MARTA (Metropolitan Atlanta Rapid Transit Authority) into DeKalb County.

In 1973 he rolled his wheelchair into a room in Piedmont Hospital to pay a visit to another person with a spinal cord injury—James Shepherd—and the visit marked the beginning of what James has called "one of the most unique and rewarding friendships I have ever shared."

It was Clark who encouraged James to go to Craig Hospital in Denver for his rehabilitation, and it was with Clark that James, upon his return, had the earliest conversations about the need for a spinal cord injury rehabilitation hospital in Atlanta.

Clark was not only an original board member, but remained one of Shepherd's most vocal, visible, and energetic boosters. After learning to fly at age 55, he piloted his plane, "The Spirit of Shepherd," solo to Alaska in 1985 to raise money for the center. A second fundraising flight—to Germany in 1987—ended in a crash-landing along the coast of Greenland, but Clark survived to tell the tale. Though he fully enjoyed his many unlikely adventures, Clark also confessed to a deeper motive: "I hope some of these newly-injured kids at Shepherd will look at me and think, 'If that old man can do these things, maybe I can too.'"

"Clark Harrison left us many things," remarked James Shepherd. "But I believe the most impressive gift Clark had to give was himself. He always gave of his time, energy, and love. Those who were lucky enough to be among Clark's friends have been truly blessed."

Reinoehl, director of nursing, "and then help with placing them in real jobs, both during the program and afterward, when they return to their hometowns."

In 1990, while concrete mixers poured foundations and huge cranes hoisted girders into the sky, Shepherd Spinal Center celebrated its fifteenth birthday. A week of festivities marked the occasion, including Volunteer Day, "Come As You Were in 1975" Day, Old-Timers Day, and Patients' Day. Shepherd's "old-timer" physicians—Dr. David Apple, Dr. Bruce Green, and Dr. Herndon Murray—were honored for 15 years of service.

It was also a time to reflect upon and reaffirm Shepherd's cardinal virtues: the family atmosphere that fosters close-knit, caring relationships between patients and staff; the team concept of rehabilitation; and the commitment to treating the whole person.

"The term 'rehabilitation' means to restore to former capacity," Dr. Apple said at the time. "At Shepherd, we take that to mean not just physical rehabilitation, but all other aspects of a person's life as well. As we enter the '90s, we are using an ever-widening circle of specialty areas to address the whole person."

What has set Shepherd apart and propelled it to the forefront of spinal injury hospitals? "Expertise and depth of services," said James Shepherd during the fifteenth-year retrospective. "I think of it as 'one-stop shopping.' We are one of the very few Model spinal cord injury programs where you get everything you need under one roof—physical rehabilitation and medical care, vocational counseling, emotional support, driver's training, everything."

Of course, what would set Shepherd apart was the $23 million expansion, and Director of Development Dell Sikes reported in mid-year that the capital campaign had already raised $10.7 million of its target of $12 million. Campaign chairman Bernie Marcus expressed confidence that the goal was within reach, especially in light of Shepherd's reputation in the community.

New medical initiatives during 1990 promised to abet that rebuilding process. First came the news from the National Institute of Neurological Disorders that a new steroid treatment could reduce paralysis significantly if administered within eight hours of injury. The drug, methylprednisolone, was reported to restore some feeling and movement in virtually all spinal cord injury patients who received it in time. Protocol for the new treatment was in place at Shepherd immediately after the news was announced. "This offers new hope to our patients," said Dr. Apple, "but it also underscores the importance of early treatment in an appropriate setting"—like Shepherd Spinal Center.

Also on the medical front, Shepherd's Dr. Brian Gill was among the researchers studying a new treatment for spasticity, a condition commonly affecting

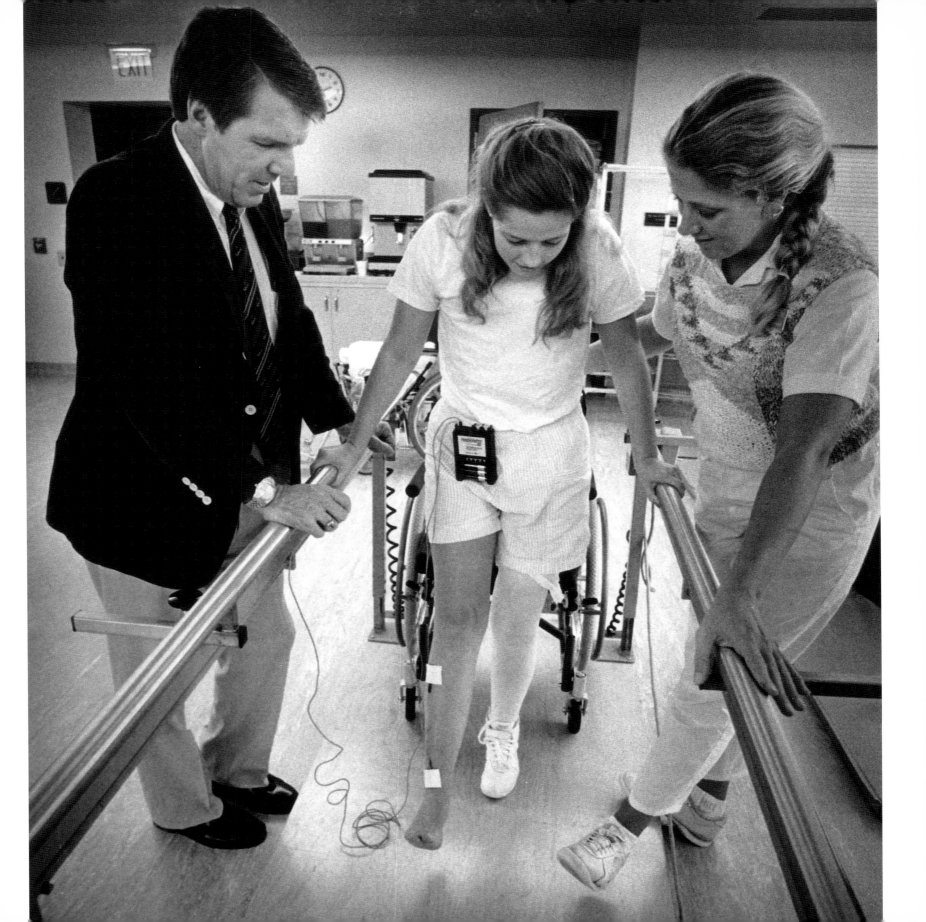

those with spinal cord injury. The treatment, called "intrathecal baclofen," works by releasing the medication (the baclofen) directly into the fluid surrounding the spinal cord, instead of taking it orally, making the medicine effective in much smaller doses. The wonderful news, according to Dr. Gill, was that more than 90 percent of the patients who had tried the treatment reported dramatic decreases in their spasticity.

Looking beyond its patients' immediate medical needs, Shepherd also implemented a new substance abuse program. "Emotional adjustment to a spinal cord injury is challenging," says Jill Koval, Ph.D., a Shepherd psychologist who helps administer the program today. "Anyone who has such an injury is at risk for turning to drugs or alcohol for self-medication and escape from the physical and emotional pain associated with life changes that accompany these injuries."

Yet another sign of Shepherd's continued growth and institutional maturity was the hiring in this milestone year of Jason Shelnutt as the center's first CFO. Jason, formerly a CPA with Pannell Kerr Forster, had been advising Shepherd on financial matters ever since he worked on the feasibility study for the new Peachtree Road facility in the early '80s and so was well prepared to assume his duties when the new position was created. (Also an ex-officio member of Shepherd's board of directors, Jason has since been promoted to Vice President for Operations, leaving the CFO's desk to Steve Holleman.)

Inside Shepherd Spinal Center and outside, people with disabilities had reason to cheer in 1990. The long-awaited Americans with Disabilities Act (ADA) was at last signed into law by congress. With its protections against discrimination in employment, transportation, public accommodations, and telecommunications, the new law emphatically guaranteed to people with disabilities their right to pursue lives of opportunity, challenge, and reward. According to SSC's advocacy specialist Mark Johnson, the law's provisions would be effected within 18 months to two years after the signing.

The following year, 1991, began with the welcome news that Shepherd had once again been named a "Model Spinal Cord Injury Program." This special designation, awarded by the U.S. Department of Education's National Institute on Disability and Rehabilitation Research (NIDRR), was bestowed upon only 13 hospitals in the country, confirming Shepherd's status among the nation's elite spinal cord injury centers. The selection also meant that Shepherd's research grant from the Institute would be funded for another five years, totaling $1.8 million.

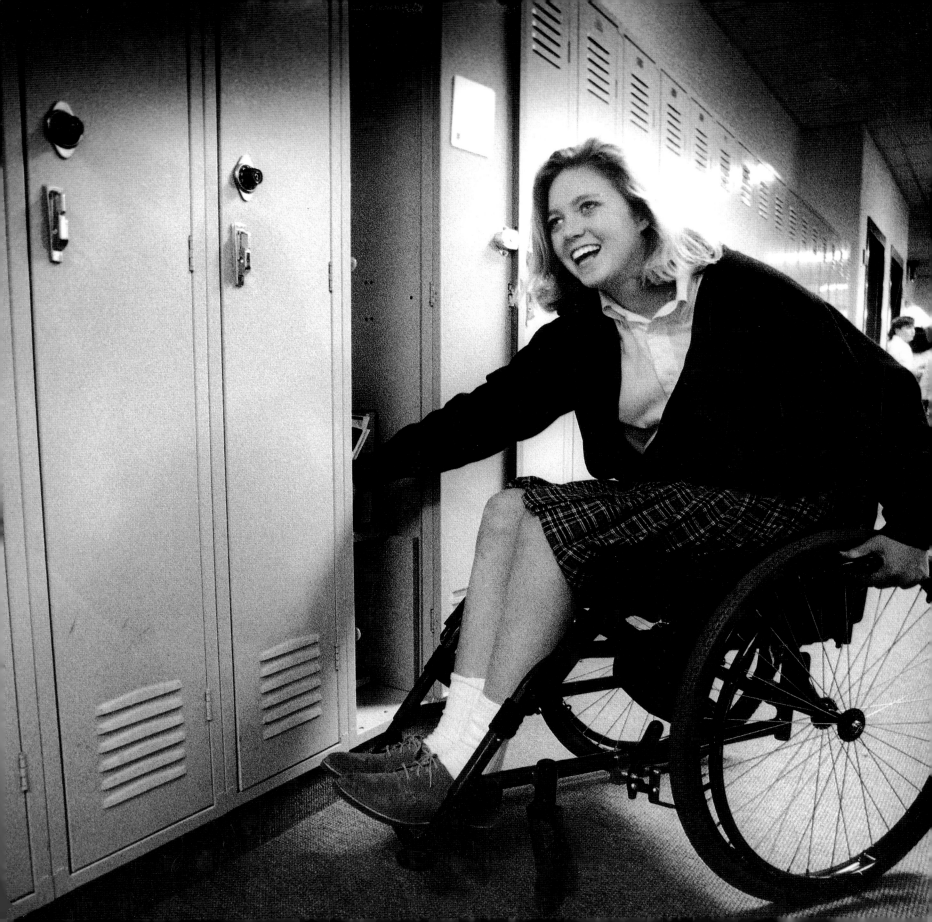

Advocacy

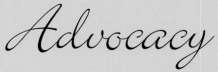

"He's one of the reasons I came here. You won't find many hospitals that will support that position."

That's Shepherd president and CEO Gary R. Ulicny, Ph.D., talking about Mark Johnson, Shepherd's advocacy coordinator, who already had been working at Shepherd for seven years when Gary arrived in 1994.

Injured in a diving accident in 1971, Mark began to get involved in advocacy during his own rehabilitation in Charlotte, North Carolina, and then he and his wife moved to Denver, where he helped found ADAPT (American Disabled for Accessible Public Transit) —"the more radical element of the disability movement." Mark and his family, including a daughter by this time, then came to Atlanta, returning to the South where both his and his wife's families lived.

His association with Shepherd began serendipitously. "In the spring of 1987 I had organized a demonstration in front of the old MARTA offices downtown, and suddenly here come all these Shepherd vehicles loaded with people ready for a march and rally. Actually, we had already won our victory in a committee vote, so it turned into a celebration of the change in MARTA policy. Later that summer, Lesley Hudson contacted me. She said, 'We like what you do. Why don't you come over here and work for us.'"

Mark doesn't need a lot of encouragement. At that MARTA protest, he says, "We had already won, so we didn't need to be disruptive. But in '89, when we hosted the national meeting of ADAPT, trying to get ADA passed without any watering down of the transit provisions, we took over the Federal Building on Spring Street and slept there all night." And he remembers with a chuckle the protest at the Greyhound Bus Depot during the same year. "Mrs. Shepherd said, 'Yes, go, but don't wear your Shepherd Spinal Center t-shirt, don't pass out business cards, and don't expect bail money.'"

Well versed in the movement's history, Mark relishes the fact Shepherd Center's 25th birthday coincides with the 25th anniversary of the passage of IDEA (Individuals with Disabilities Education Act). "It's a great irony that at the same time Shepherd was being founded, parents of kids with disabilities were coming together to insist that their kids be able to go to neighborhood schools. Their work resulted in the 1975 legislation mandating the right of these kids to an appropriate mainstream education."

And, of course, the year 2000 also marks the tenth anniversary of the passage of the ADA, and Mark has been at the forefront of the effort to "Renew the Pledge." At a conference three years ago in Oregon, Mark recalls, "we formed a group called Initiative 2000, whose mission was to create a number of awareness-raising events that would foster renewed support and dedication to the provisions of the ADA as its tenth anniversary approached." The three-year effort culminated in the nationally publicized cross-country Spirit of ADA Torch Relay, which swept through Atlanta—and Shepherd Center—on July 20 and 21, on its way to Washington, D.C, and, finally, New York City.

For Mark, the event meant more than great PR. "The number of attacks on ADA has been increasing in the past couple of years," he says. "Of course, that's because we keep pushing harder for implementation."

Mark intends to keep pushing, and he expects that Shepherd will help him. "What I like about Shepherd is that it has the determination to move forward with the agenda, but also the flexibility to find a pace that doesn't hurt too bad—that doesn't alienate people and ultimately backfire."

"Consistent designation as a Model Center means that what we are doing works," said Dr. Apple, who directs the federal award project. "Aggressive rehabilitation programs, combined with a holistic approach, have kept Shepherd on the cutting edge."

The good news continued with word from the development department that the capital campaign's goal of raising $12 million for the new expansion had been surpassed. By spring, $12.7 in gifts and pledges had been received, thanks to the untiring efforts of campaign chairman Bernie Marcus, along with Emory Schwall, chairman of the Individuals and Foundations Committee; Harald Hansen, chairman of the Corporate Committee; Fred Alias, campaign vice chairman; and board members Alana and James Shepherd.

A related celebration occurred on June 20, when members of the board of directors, the advisory board, and the administration joined with the staff of Holder Construction (builders of the new expansion) for a "topping out" ceremony. Once it had been officially signed by all the guests and construction crew members, the traditional white beam was hoisted into place at the top of the new building's steel superstructure. Tangible evidence that "the best was yet to come."

Strengthening its commitment to the wider community of people with disabilities, Shepherd worked hard in 1991 to bring "independent living" closer to reality for people unable to manage on their own. With funding from Shepherd, former quadriplegic patient Jenny Langley began a 12-month experimental program wherein she would receive the full-time attendant care that would enable her to live independently at her home rather than in a nursing home or other institutional setting. The success of the program would demonstrate to the Georgia legislature that people with disabilities could live independent and fulfilling lives without undue burden upon taxpayers.

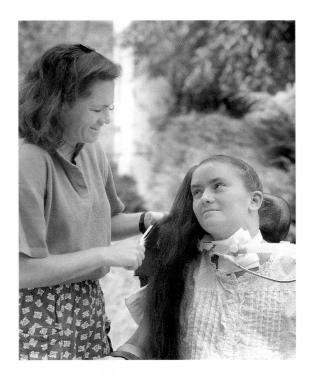

According to advocacy specialist Mark Johnson, "The government mandates nursing home care, not attendant services, though the costs are similar. . . . Most of the money flows to institutions, not the individuals who need it." Thanks to Shepherd and to the pilot program with Jenny Langley, legislators began to see the light. The state of Georgia allocated $150,000 for attendant services in fiscal year '92. "It's a start," said Mark.

With the rising cost of medical care—and of insurance—the affordability of attendant care was but one of many financial issues exerting increasing pressure upon SSC. In a nutshell, Shepherd found itself providing more care to more people without adequate means to pay for it. As Dell Sikes noted, Shepherd was providing "millions of dollars of uncompensated care to these patients each year." But Dell was also announcing the beginnings of a solution to the problem. In 1991, with a specially earmarked gift from the Auxiliary in the amount of

$32,000, Shepherd's Patient Care Endowment Fund was officially established. With a target fund balance of $5 million by 1995, the endowment would provide a self-sustaining source of income so Shepherd could always continue to serve patients with limited financial resources.

Continuing at the forefront of technological advance, Shepherd was one of 20 rehabilitation centers across the country involved in the 1991 research trial of Parastep I, a system of "functional electrical stimulation" (FES) designed to simulate the walking function in people with certain levels of paraplegia. According to Dr. Donald P. Leslie, director of Shepherd's outpatient department and lead physician on the project, "Electrical stimulation is one area where we see a lot of promising work being done." Shepherd enlisted 10 patients in the project, the potential benefits of which would be strengthening of weakened muscles and, ideally, at least some wheelchair-free mobility. Eleven months later Myrtice Atrice, the physical therapist working with Dr. Leslie on the project, reported that most of the patients testing the system were walking at least 50 to 150 feet.

Another important test was underway at Shepherd at the same time. The physical therapy department began conducting a unique five-year research program into the benefits of cardiovascular fitness for people rehabilitating from spinal cord injury or disease. With medical advances lengthening the lives of the spinal cord injured, the issue of physical fitness was coming to the fore, and the Shepherd study was the first in the nation to look long-term (up to two years post-injury) at patients' fitness and the relation between fitness and function. According to physical therapist Sarah Morrison, "Over time, we expect to see weight shifts, transfers, and pushing endurance to improve because of a healthier heart, stronger muscles, and lower weight gain."

Fitness certainly had its day on July 4, 1991, with the tenth running of the Wheelchair Division of the Peachtree Road Race. Craig Blanchette (who had also won in '87 and '89) attributed his record-shattering win to being "in the best shape I've been in in two years." SSC recreation therapist Stacy Green, who took over directorship of the race from original coordinator Barb Trader (formerly Barb Leidheiser), agreed that the athletes' "rigorous training schedules" explained this year's faster times. As testimony to the Wheelchair Division's growing national prestige, 1991 was the first year it was funded completely through private support. Volkswagen United States, in its second year of sponsorship, led the way with a $20,000 donation.

Before the year was out, and with a look at the next year looming, the new Art Selection Committee, chaired by Carolyn Caswell, took on the job of locating artworks to adorn the new building—scheduled for completion in April. "On the road back to independence," said committee member Alana Shepherd, "the hallways of Shepherd will be one of the most important 'art tours' our patients ever make."

The Ascent of the Phoenix (Society)

"It's always nice to see college girls at the spinal center," remarked a patient during the summer of 1980. He was talking about the debutantes of The Phoenix Society of Atlanta, who during that summer 20 years ago adopted Shepherd Spinal Center as the beneficiary of their volunteer efforts, and who have been brightening the corridors ever since.

In addition to volunteering at the center—a minimum of 18 hours each—the Phoenix debs also held their first organized event that year: a Dance-a-Thon at the home of Mr. and Mrs. Ralph Toon. The girls secured sponsors for each hour danced and proceeded to raise several thousand dollars for the new building fund. In 1981 the debs put on a Skate-a-Thon that raised another $5,000, and a tradition was firmly entrenched.

In 1984 came the first Grits at the Ritz, a brunch and fashion show which served both to honor the summer-long volunteer efforts of the debs and to raise additional money for Shepherd. For the first seven years of this now 16-year-old annual event, fashions were supplied by Neiman Marcus. Since that time a variety of clothiers and jewelers have generously contributed their time and effort.

But the real time and effort comes from the Phoenix debs themselves, who over the years have volunteered in every effort imaginable. In addition to the day-to-day tasks of helping with meals and patient outings, answering phones in ICU, and manning the gift shop and information desk, the young women have created a number of special patient parties—Christmas in July, South of the Border, and The Psychedelic '60's, to name a few. In the early '90s, the Wheelchair Division of the Peachtree Road Race became a special focus of the debs' efforts, and since that time the Phoenix Society debs have been a mainstay of volunteer effort for this huge annual event.

At the Grits at the Ritz celebration in 1988, Taryn Chilivis was honored for 66 hours of summer volunteer work, a record achievement at the time. But two years later Taryn's record was smashed by Melinda Douglas, who remains the all-time Phoenix volunteer champion with 125 hours of service.

Other members of the Phoenix Society's volunteer pantheon include:

Debbie Johnson, 1991

Sharri Teel, 1992

Susan Warren, 1993

Cassandra Martin, 1994

Danielle Babcock, 1995

Holli Austin and Paige Younkins, 1996

Noush Leahy, 1997

Mary Elizabeth Rozema, 1998

Ramsey Burke, 1999

Amanda Kaye Ellenburg, 2000

Over 20 years, these and all the members of the Phoenix Society have helped raise countless thousands of dollars for the benefit of Shepherd Center. More important, they have given the most valuable gift of all—themselves—and become an integral part of the volunteer spirit that makes Shepherd such a unique institution.

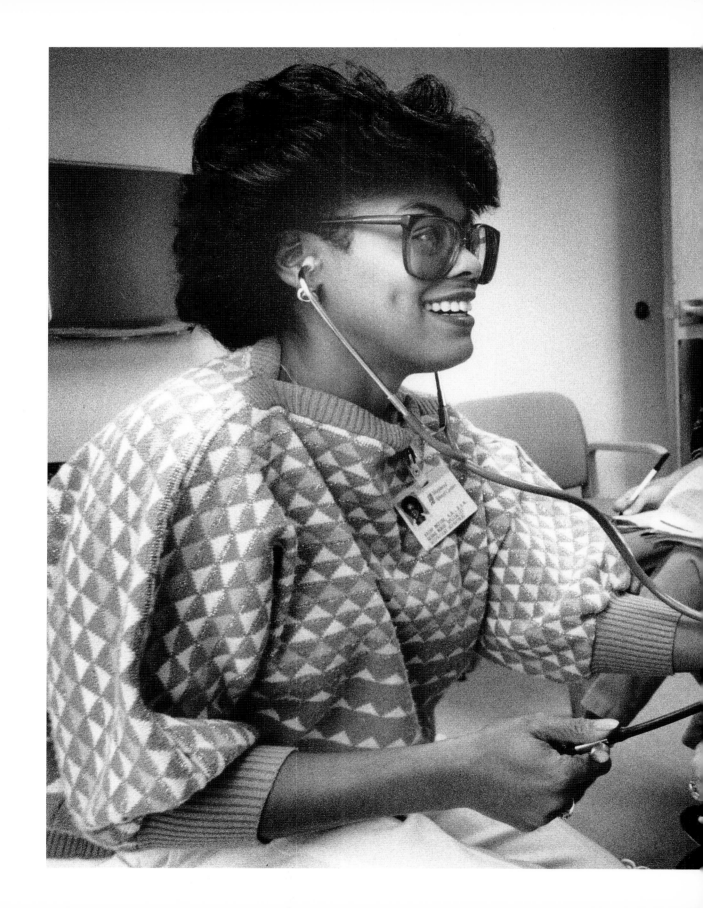

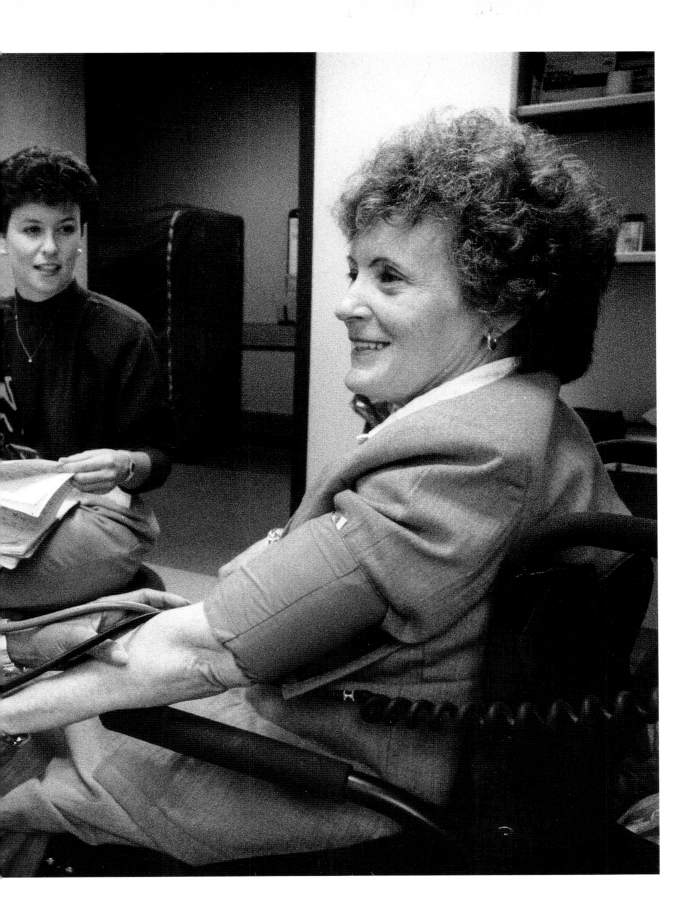

The Best is Here

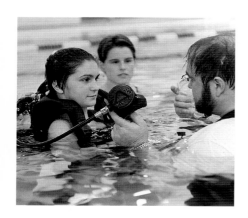

On May 13, 1992, 10 years to the day after Shepherd Spinal Center moved into its own facility on Peachtree Road, the "new expansion" celebrated its grand opening—and, at long last, its christening. At the gala dedication ceremony, Bernie Marcus, who had successfully chaired the capital campaign, surprised his wife, Billi, with the ultimate birthday present—an artist's rendering of the new structure revealing its official name: The Billi Marcus Building. The naming honored Mrs. Marcus's many contributions to Shepherd over the years, especially her dedicated chairmanship of The RTM Challenge, an event that in four years had raised more than a half-million dollars.

Then came the evening's second surprise. Mr. Marcus presented to Alana Shepherd $4 million in The Home Depot stock, $3 million to go toward construction costs and $1 million to establish the Billi and Bernie Marcus Patient Care Endowment Fund.

The celebration also featured a keynote address by U.S. Senator Max Cleland (then Georgia's Secretary of State), who proclaimed Shepherd "the finest rehabilitation center for spinal cord injury in the nation," and the official ribbon-cutting ceremony, performed by two of Shepherd's young patients—12-year-old Chrissie Stahl and four-year-old Shaqueshia Powell.

Touring the new facility during the Grand Opening, guests were especially wowed by the new state-of-the-art therapeutic recreation center. Among its world-class features: an aquatic center with a 25-yard pool offering, among other things, hydro-aquatics, swimming lessons, and SCUBA certification; a full-court gymnasium with an elevated indoor track; a weight room fully equipped for a complete strengthening program; and an arts and crafts suite offering woodworking, pottery, a photography darkroom, and areas for painting, drawing, and other creative activities. The complex would also house Shepherd's new fitness center, ProMotion, designed to be totally wheelchair accessible and open not only to the hospital's patients and staff, but to the community at large.

While doubling the size of Shepherd Spinal Center as a whole, the new building gave special attention to the needs of the ever-expanding outpatient

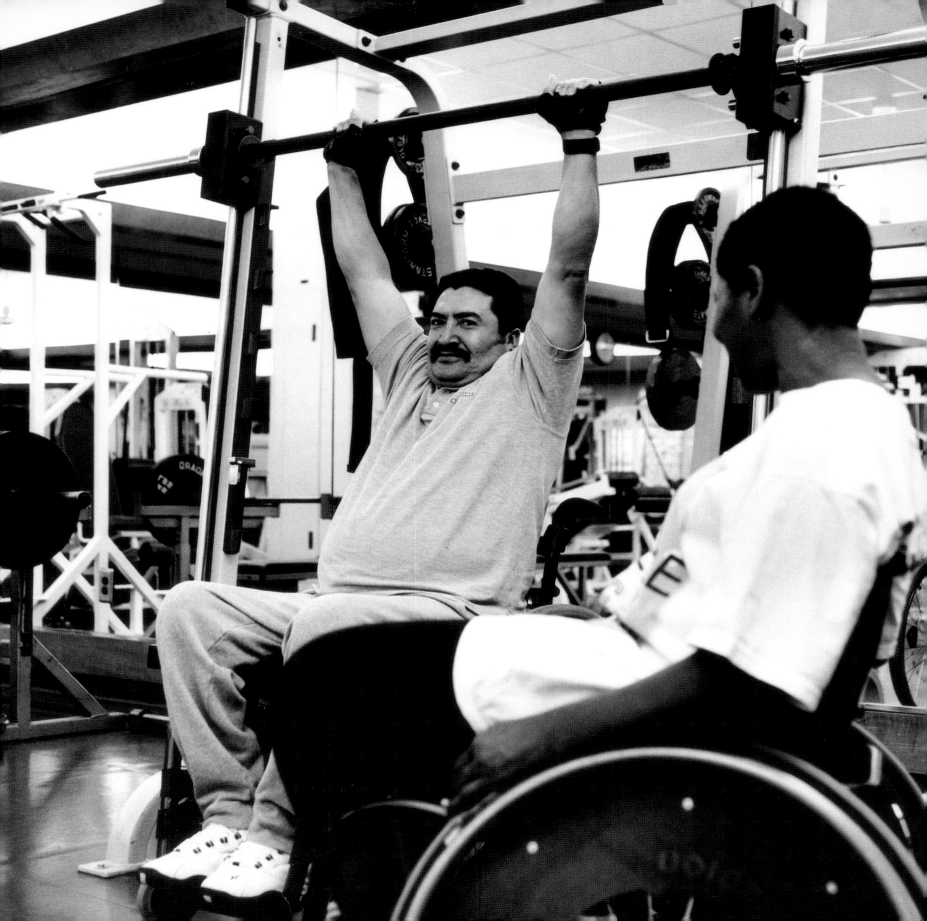

department. With eight times the space it occupied previously, the department now included a pharmacy, ten examination rooms, a therapy gym, two separate therapy rooms, a transitional living lab, and a separate waiting area. "We certainly have a world-class physical plant now," proclaimed Dr. Donald P. Leslie, medical director of outpatient services.

The expanded outpatient facilities also allowed for the continued growth and development of new programs, services, and specialty clinics—including Dr. Leslie's post-polio syndrome clinic, which has steadily grown to provide an invaluable service to a very special patient population. "I went to the University of Michigan," says Dr. Leslie, "and studied under Frederick Maynard, now the guru of polio, and we modeled our program after his. I regard polio as a spinal cord injury, in effect, because it attacks the cells that give the spinal cord its muscular capabilities. Post-polio patients are a great population, a challenging population, and we're seeing more and more of them—probably 30 a year. In fact, we're now the home of the monthly meeting of the Atlanta Post-Polio Association."

Shepherd's recently opened Multiple Sclerosis (MS) Center was also well positioned to take advantage of the new space. According to former medical director Dr. William H. Stuart, the Multiple Sclerosis Center at Shepherd was the result of a fortuitous set of circumstances. Dr. Stuart, who had been treating a substantial number of MS patients in his private practice and who saw the need for a comprehensive MS center in Atlanta, originally approached Piedmont Hospital with the idea. "They liked the concept," says Dr. Stuart, "but didn't want to fund it. At the same time, though, the MS Society was approaching Shepherd with the idea of creating a center. Shepherd turned to Piedmont for a partner in the undertaking, and of course Piedmont was already aware of my interest. For a while it looked like the center would in fact be a collaboration between Shepherd and Piedmont. But Piedmont ultimately declined, and Shepherd very graciously stepped forward to take the project on."

Consequently, immediately upon its inception, the MS Center at Shepherd was designated by the National Multiple Sclerosis Society as the only comprehensive center of its type in the Southeast. With no known cause and therefore no cure for this disabling neurological disorder, the stated goal of the MS program was to slow the progress of the disease and to focus on a rehabilitation program that emphasized a lifestyle of maximum independence. But the physicians sensed that a revolution in MS care was afoot, and they planned to help foment it.

In fact, on October 21, just a few months after moving into its new quarters, the MS Center at Shepherd hosted an open house to celebrate its first-year anniversary and to highlight its comprehensive, cutting-edge program. The latest

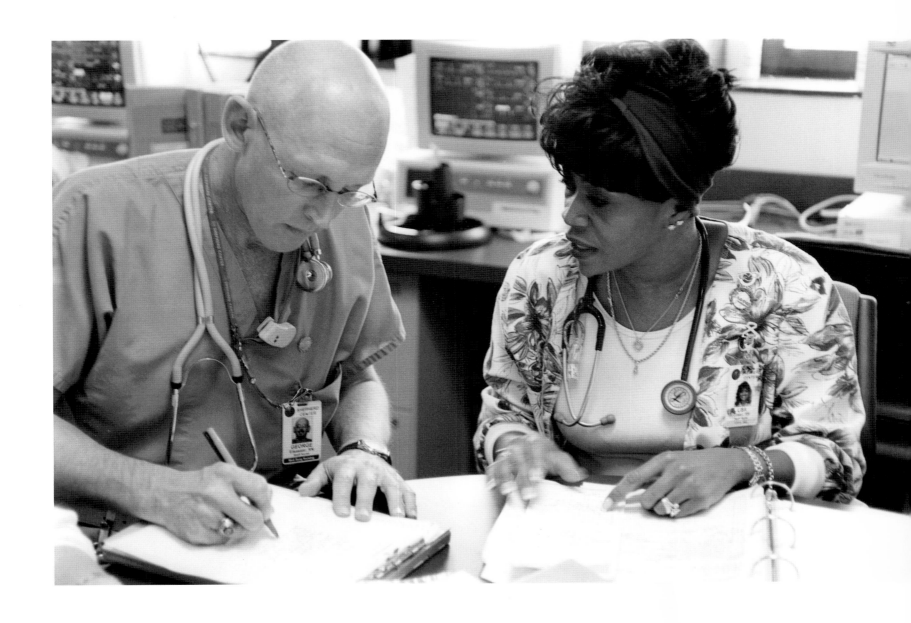

technology—cooling vests, balance trainers, the new MRI (Magnetic Resonance Imaging) laboratory—was on display, along with presentations from both the Georgia Chapter and the National Multiple Sclerosis Society. Of particular note, at just one year old, the MS Center at Shepherd had treated more than 300 patients and was serving approximately 30 new patients each month.

Our very sudden growth was actually a shock to everyone. We have to credit the hard work of our first staffers, Peggy Brown (director, outpatient services

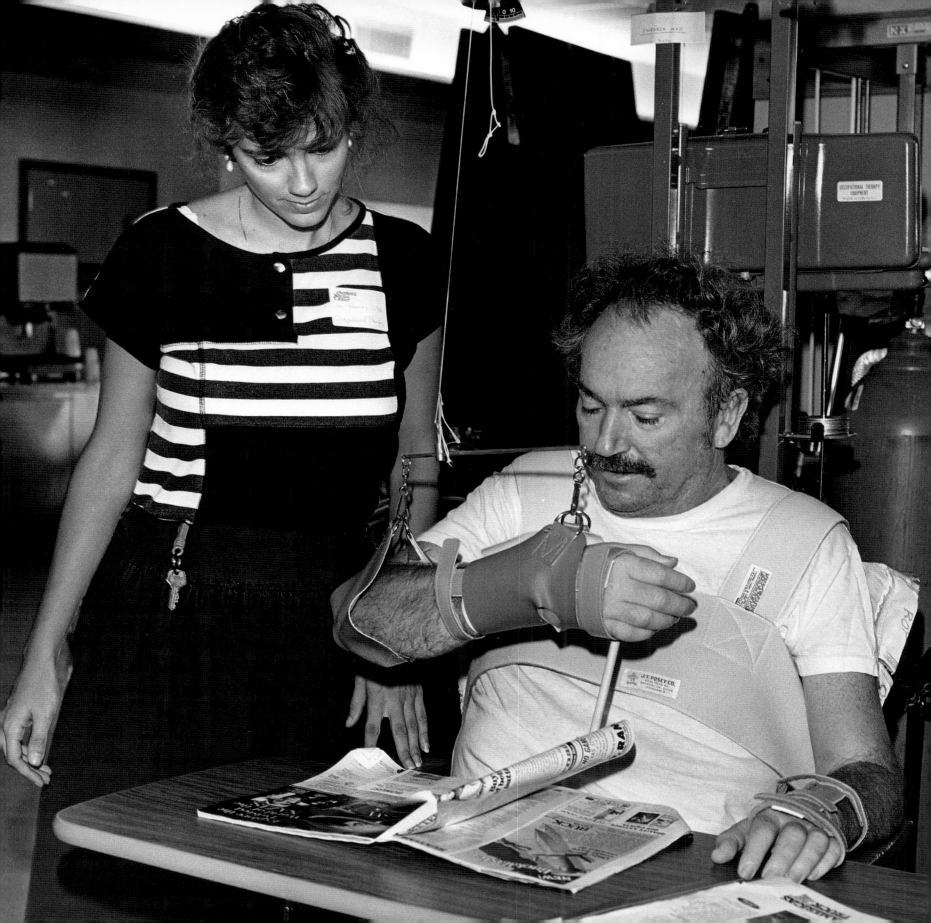

and MS Center) and Ismari "Issi" Clesson (then manager, MS Center), who were amazingly dedicated people. But the center's growth was largely attributable to the staff's ability to shape the program to address the real needs of the patients. We originally envisioned a few hundred patients coming to us primarily to address their rehabilitative needs. But we ended up with thousands of patients coming to us for something quite different: they wanted us to do something to modify the rate of their illness. It was time to revise our model.

Meanwhile, inside the Shepherd Building, the urology department was experiencing equally dramatic growth. Dr. James Bennett and Dr. Jenelle Foote had joined Dr. Bruce Green's medical staff, and the department had expanded to offer three distinct, though closely related, services.

In the continence clinic, able-bodied and people with disabilities experiencing this often embarrassing condition could find "the latest expertise in the treatment of incontinence," according to Dr. Green. The available treatments ranged from the simple "bladder drill" (i.e., carefully following an individualized urination schedule) to various types of reconstructive surgery. "Reconstructive urology," says Dr. Green today, "in which we enlarge the bladder using parts of the patient's intestine, is one of the most important advances we've seen in the treatment of incontinence."

The male fertility clinic—ongoing since 1987—expanded its work with men who wanted to become fathers but who were unable to ejaculate because of neurological impairment—whether from spinal cord injury or related conditions. Among the clinic's advanced treatment options were vibromassage, electroejaculation stimulation (EES), and in vitro fertilization (IVF). "The process requires much patience and a big commitment from patients and family members," says Dr. Green, "but the benefits are considerable."

(Over the next year, in fact, two of SSC's own would enjoy those benefits. Stacy Green, then a supervisor in the therapeutic recreation department and director of the Wheelchair Division of the Peachtree Road Race, and her husband Jimmy, a wheelchair racer and former Shepherd patient, availed themselves of the clinic's in vitro fertilization procedure, and Stacy not only became pregnant but delivered twins, Caitlyn and Nathan Green. Coincidentally, Barb Trader, then director of therapeutic recreation (and Stacy's supervisor) discovered that she too was pregnant after she and husband Scott Holland had been through Shepherd's fertility program.)

And finally, males suffering from impotence were finding a variety of successful treatments—and new hope for sexual intimacy—in the urology department's erectile dysfunction clinic. According to Dr. Bennett, "At Shepherd we have been very successful with a variety of treatment possibilities for neurological impotence"—including advances in pharmacology (like today's Viagra), new non-surgical devices, and implant surgery. Looking down the road, Dr. Green

The Shepherds—both James and Alana—have been totally supportive of me in anything I wanted to try, even the most innovative things. We've never been turned down or discouraged from moving ahead and staying ahead.

—Dr. Bruce Green
Medical Director,
Urology Department

sees drugs like Viagra as exemplifying a promising development—i.e., the growing use of non-invasive procedures rather than surgery. "When the clinic started," he says, "just about all we could offer was penile implants, which, over time, tended to cause complications in spinal cord injured males. Now we have Viagra, injection therapy, and other less invasive procedures with better results. And we're now doing very little implant surgery."

The year's big news—the opening of The Billi Marcus Building—had been four years in the making. Ironically, another exciting story, whose first chapter was being written now in 1992, would come to its dramatic culmination in 1996. Thanks greatly to the efforts of Shepherd Spinal Center board members, staff, and friends—several of whom traveled to Tigne, France, to formally present the city's bid, Atlanta was chosen as the site of the 1996 Paralympic Games.

But it wasn't easy. Those who assumed that the Paralympics would inevitably take place in the Olympics host city were quickly disabused. "It was a tough fight to get the Paralympics here," recalls Alana Shepherd, "a fight that we fought with dignity. In fact, the Atlanta Committee for the Olympic Games (ACOG) wanted no part of the event. Of course, they were scared of it, didn't understand it, and already had all they could handle. So unless we stepped up, it wasn't going to happen."

Mark Johnson, Shepherd's advocacy specialist and one of the games' early supporters, remembers those days vividly: "All of us had hoped that Billy Payne, head of the Atlanta Committee for the Olympic Games, would naturally include the Paralympics as part of Atlanta's bid, and at an early meeting down at Georgia Tech, some of our therapeutic recreation staff approached him about it. But he saw it as a glob-on. 'We have momentum now, we have a chance . . . I can't be bothered with that.' That was his attitude. After Atlanta got the games, our group returned and said, 'Will you help us now? It would be terrible, especially in Atlanta with its civil rights history, for the Paralympics to be spurned.' But Billy again said, 'Go away. Don't bother me.' That's when Alana Shepherd and Harald Hansen took over."

When July brought the first official visit from International Paralympic Committee (IPC) members, again SSC was front and center. The four representatives rode in the lead vehicle of the eleventh annual Wheelchair Division of the Peachtree Road Race and were hosted by members of Shepherd's board of directors. The 1996 Paralympics would be the first time the United States had hosted an international event for disabled athletes of such magnitude, and Shepherd would make it happen.

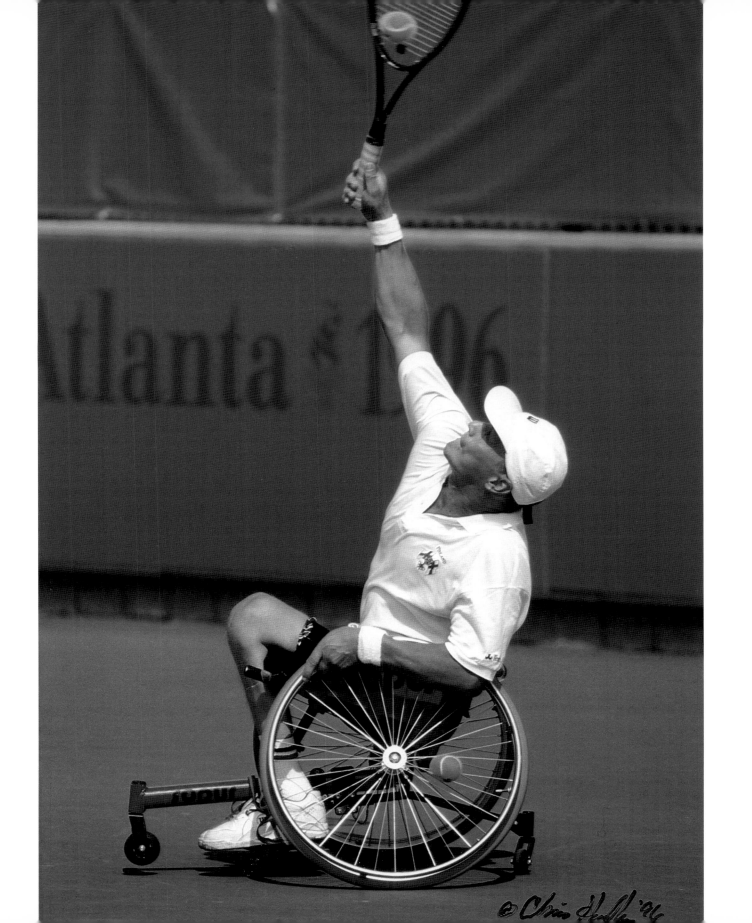

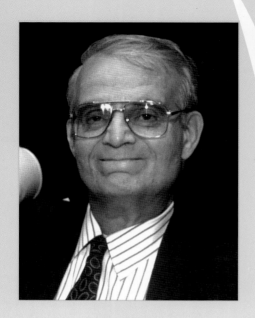

In Memorium:
David Webb
(d. August 28, 1992)

"As soon as we began talking about starting a spinal center," says James Shepherd, "David Webb's name came up—a community leader who was enjoying a very full and successful life despite a disability—obviously somebody we needed to talk to. We met for lunch, and when we asked him if he wanted to join the dream, he was on board immediately."

Native Atlantan David Webb was injured after his junior year at Northside High School at a first-of-summer pool party. He was diving through an inner tube—"something I'd done hundreds of times," as he pointed out—but this time his head hit the tube and the impact bruised his spinal cord.

Following his injury, Dave graduated from Northside and searched for a wheelchair accessible college in the area. Upon discovering there was no such thing, he enrolled at Emory University because it suited his career goal of becoming an attorney. He stayed on for law school and passed the bar exam before graduating.

All of the law firms to which he applied declined to hire him, but Harold Patterson, general counsel of the Federal Reserve Bank, offered him a job, and Dave spent the first 10 years of his career there. In 1972, the Trust Company of Georgia (now SunTrust Bank) decided to start its own legal department and hired Dave to head it up. He spent the rest of his career as Trust Company's corporate counsel.

Dave met Carmen Rodrigues, who was attending Georgia State University on a Rotary International Scholarship, in 1975, and they were married the following year.

In addition to serving as one of Shepherd's founding board members, Dave was the chairman of Jimmy Carter's White House Conference on Handicapped Individuals, a board member of the National Paraplegia Foundation, and a director of the Georgia Easter Seals Society. In 1974 he was named one of the Jaycees "Ten Outstanding Young Men in America."

Dave's own words best put this remarkable life in perspective: "A disabled person must do the best he can with what he's got. In spite of being disabled—even severely disabled—life can and must be an extremely exciting adventure."

Before the year drew to a close, Shepherd was the beneficiary of two unique and generous gifts. In memory of her mother, Frances D. Wagenhals, Ms. Lois Sanders donated a one-bedroom condominium to the center, to be used by the families of patients undergoing rehabilitation at Shepherd. Also, the new gynecology clinic (another part of the expanded outpatient department) received a donation from outpatient Margaret Staton, who herself had been paralyzed most of her life due to a spinal tumor. Ms. Staton, who would later serve as a member of both the board of directors and the advisory board, stipulated that her gift benefit women who would not otherwise be able to afford gynecological services, and she pledged additional gifts to assist the clinic.

The Billi Marcus Building remained in sharp focus the following year, as patients and staff continued to seize upon—and marvel at—the opportunities for growth and enhancement afforded by the new space.

It could be argued, though, that of all the programs and services that were dramatically enhanced by the opening of the Marcus Building, none benefited more than the MS Center. With its designation as the only official multiple sclerosis center in the Southeast, its complete range of cutting-edge treatments and technology, and its expert—and expanding—medical team, the MS Center at Shepherd was becoming increasingly aggressive in its battle against this disorder. And the center's vision of a revolution in MS care was being realized: We now viewed MS as a treatable disease, and our medical team began treating it more vigorously.

At the same time, Dr. Robert Gilbert, explained in detail why Shepherd's MS patients had reason to be encouraged: "Before, MS patients had to go to 10 different places for different facets of treatment. The beauty of the MS Center at Shepherd is that we have everything—neurology, neuroimaging, psychology, urology, nursing and all the therapies—under one roof. There are very few places in the country like this."

Furthermore, on the pharmacology front, 1993 brought FDA approval for the production of beta interferon, one of the first drugs demonstrated to slow the progression of MS. Coincidentally, Dr. Douglas S. Stuart—a new member of Shepherd's MS staff—was involved in beta interferon research during his residency at the University of Chicago. "The results were compelling," he said at the time. "It's the first major breakthrough, the first effective, long-term treatment."

Outside SSC's walls, but fueled with Shepherd's enthusiasm, the Atlanta Paralympic Organizing Committee (APOC) took up the tremendous challenge of preparing to host the 1996 Paralympic Games. The prize had been secured, and, with the passing of the Paralympic flag into the hands of APOC president Andy Fleming at the closing ceremonies in Barcelona, the monumental task of readying Atlanta for the games lay ahead.

The extent to which Shepherd would be involved in that labor could be measured by a quick look at the number of SSC representatives on the committee. From the staff: Dr. David Apple, medical director of the center; Dr. Donald Leslie, associate medical director; Barb Trader, director of therapeutic recreation; and Ann Cody-Morris, SSC sports and fitness specialist and Paralympic athlete. And from the Shepherd board of directors: Harald Hansen, APOC chairman; Alana Shepherd, vice chairman; Fred Alias, Carl Knobloch, and James Shepherd. Not to mention the herculean effort that would be provided by countless additional Shepherd staff members and volunteers.

In fact, just how much work would be involved was hard to foresee, as James Shepherd recalls. "I told Harald Hansen that he could easily handle being chair of the Paralympics board, that it was only going to take part of one day each week. Maybe that was a bit naïve. But he rose to the occasion."

Barcelona had set the bar high, not only providing the 1992 Paralympic athletes with outstanding services and facilities, but also packing every venue with throngs of enthusiastic fans. But Fleming vowed that APOC would meet the challenge. "We plan to provide a complete and exciting all-around experience for the athletes," he said, meaning not only excellent housing, smooth operations, and social and recreational opportunities, but also plenty of attention from media and spectators. He had reason to expect success: "We have had a tremendous sense of community enthusiasm and support, especially from Shepherd Spinal Center."

True to its mission, Shepherd was reaching out into the larger community in another important way in 1993. Realizing that other hospitals in the region could benefit from its expertise and resources as a federally designated Model Center, Shepherd initiated the Southeastern Spinal Cord Network. According to Dr. David Apple, "The network will provide an excellent framework for the physicians at SSC to share information and work with physicians throughout the Southeast. This should enable spinal cord injured patients to receive specialized care without having to travel to Atlanta." Response to the creation of the network was immediate and enthusiastic; within a few months of its announcement, 66 health care facilities across the Southeast had contacted Shepherd to express

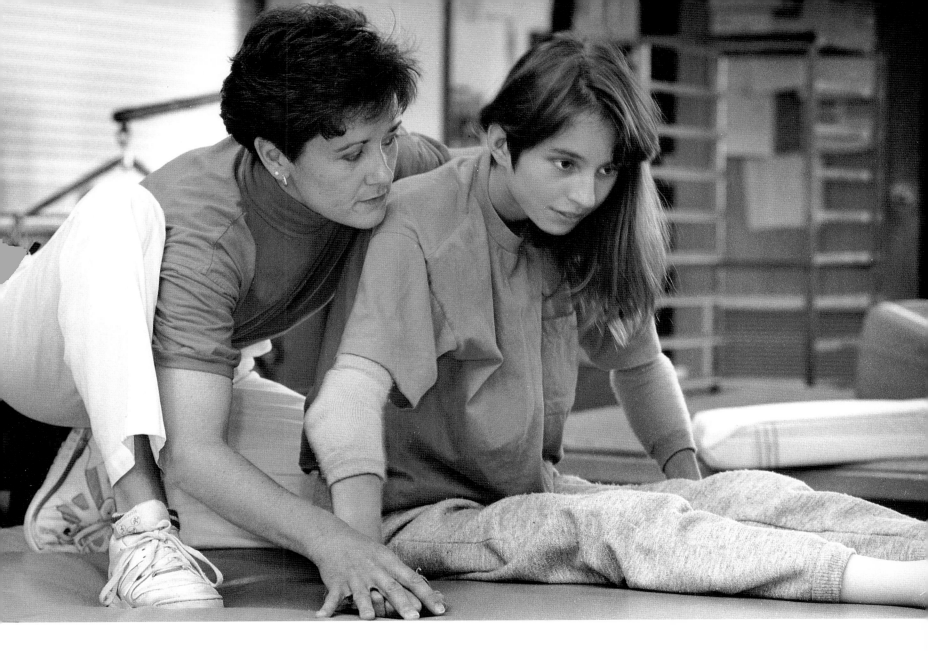

their interest. Within one year, the network had 15 full-fledged members.

Finally, 1993 brought much-deserved recognition to two of Shepherd's most loyal and generous supporters. Deen Day Smith and Bernie Marcus were recipients of the prestigious Horatio Alger Award, annually presented to 10 Americans who have overcome adversity to make outstanding contributions in their chosen fields. Both Mrs. Smith, chairman of the Cecil B. Day Investment Company, and Mr. Marcus, chairman of The Home Depot, have contributed immeasurably to Shepherd's growth and achievement.

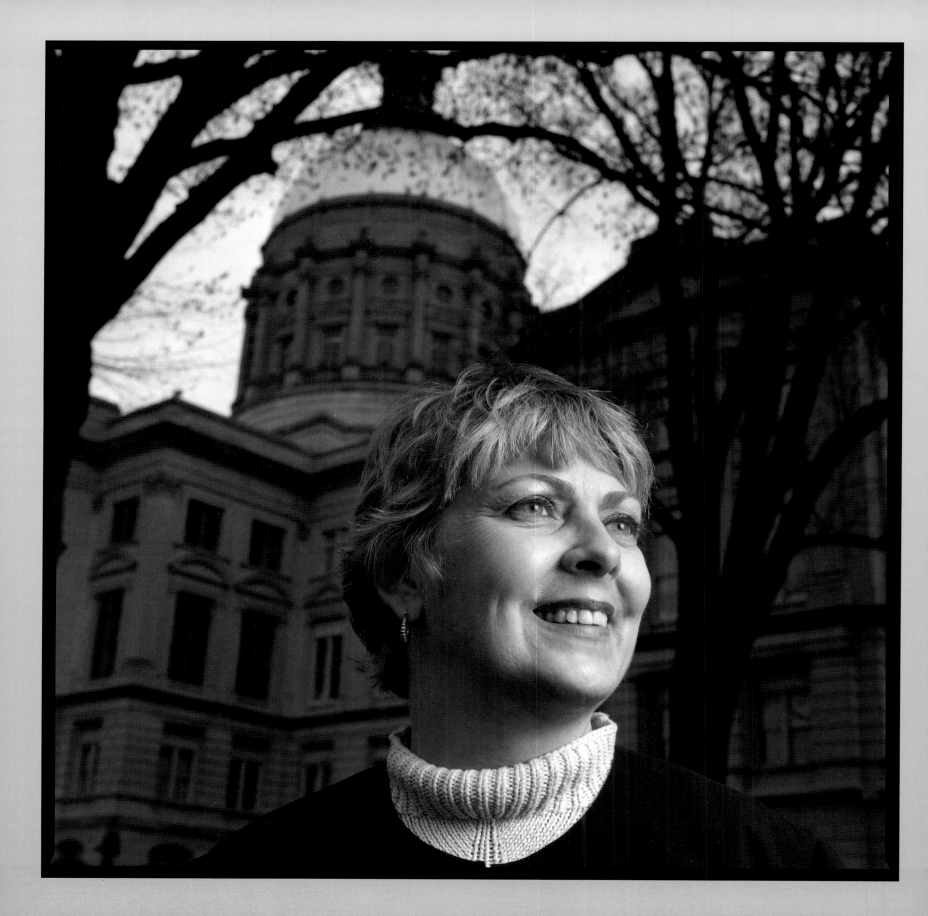

When Cindy Cutter's father, Arne Olson, became paralyzed following an operation for an aorta aneurysm, Cindy was too preoccupied with his condition to give much thought to the strange symptoms she herself was experiencing. In fact, as Mr. Olson completed his rehabilitation at Shepherd Center, Cindy's symptoms seemed to disappear.

But a year later, they resurfaced, particularly a loss of balance so severe that she couldn't walk without leaning on nearby walls for support. When her husband, Walt, insisted she seek treatment, a neurologist diagnosed her with MS. Then he sent her home, where she read every book she could find on the disease and watched her condition deteriorate.

During a family visit to Shepherd, she stopped by to say hello to Dr. Donald Leslie, who had treated her father. The moment he saw her, Dr. Leslie realized that Cindy needed to be in the care of the Multiple Sclerosis Center at Shepherd.

Today, Cindy talks frankly about how fortunate she feels. "I go to Shepherd every three months to check in," she says, "and I'm doing great. I'm taking one of the 'ABC' drugs (Avonex, Betaseron, and Copaxone), and it has made a major, major difference. Thanks to these drugs, the intensity of the exacerbations is much weaker and the duration is much shorter, so everything about the disease is diminished. Now it's more of an inconvenience, whereas it used to be more like a nightmare."

Cindy organized the first MS peer support group at Shepherd and ran it for two years, but, increasingly, advocacy on behalf of the disabled community has become her passion. "Now, instead of being a peer supporter, I go talk to different MS peer groups, to try to get them politically active. Do you realize that the largest minority in the country is people with disabilities. Imagine the pull we would have if we would all get out and vote. That's my message when I talk to these groups."

Of course, Cindy must also make time for her career — as the proprietor of Encore Properties, a commercial real estate company she started three years ago. She specializes in renovating warehouses into class-A office space and leasing it out. "It's going well," she says. "I get downtown three or four times a week, and since I'm my own boss, I can make appointments when it works best for me."

Cindy continues to spread the word about Shepherd. "I talk to lots of people with MS, and the first thing I ask them is, 'How many MS patients does your doctor treat?' They'll say, 'Oh, three or four,' and I say, 'Run. Go to Shepherd right now.'

"The thing is, with MS, I can put 10 patients in the same room, and the disease will be affecting them in totally different ways. So it's imperative that you get a doctor with lots of experience, who really knows MS."

With Shepherd's help, Cindy has dealt with her disease. And as she checks her pulse these days, she finds herself more full of life than ever. "I know this sounds strange," she says, "but I know I'm a better person now, more focused, with more meaning in my life. I have a better idea of what things are important now, what to blow off and what to take seriously. I'm a stronger person, and I'm glad."

(Thanks to Shira M. Davis's profile of Cindy, "Learning to Live with MS," Spinal Column, Spring 1993, pp. 12-14.)

Cindy Cutter

"I know this sounds strange, but I know I'm a better person now, more focused, with more meaning in my life."

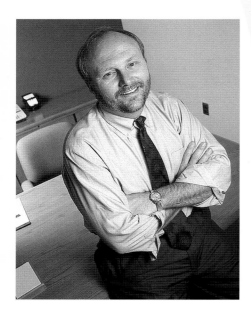

One thing I'm very proud of is that we have remained independent, instead of joining any of the health care networks, and that, instead of failing or being swallowed up, we've grown. We've created jobs.

—*Gary R. Ulicny, Ph.D.*
President and CEO

With the retirement of James B. Collins, who had been the center's administrator since the move to Peachtree Road, the lead story of 1994 became the search for and hiring of the person who would lead Shepherd into the new millennium. The search would be challenging. So would the job. As James Shepherd said at the time, "This leader will be charged with keeping the nation's most progressive rehabilitation center at the forefront of the field as we proceed through the inevitable changes brought about by health care reform."

"It was a time of great change," says Gary Ulicny now, as he looks back to his hiring in 1994 as Shepherd's first president and CEO. "I'm not sure whether I walked into it or initiated it. Shepherd's clinical skills had always been the best; its people on the floors were the best. But in some ways—especially in getting prepared for managed care—we found ourselves a little bit behind the times. We needed to make some changes."

Ulicny, who holds a Ph.D. in behavioral psychology, came to Shepherd from Raleigh, North Carolina, where he had been administrative director of rehabilitation services at the Wake Hospital System, which included a 550-bed acute care hospital and a 56-bed rehabilitation hospital. "Probably the greatest strength I bring to Shepherd," Ulicny said at the time of his hiring, "is my background administering a lot of different rehabilitation services."

In fact, shortly after taking the reins, Ulicny announced a major expansion of Shepherd's services: the center would now offer treatment for acquired brain injury (ABI). At the same time came news of an organizational overhaul: rather than being structured according to departments and disciplines, Shepherd would now operate on a "product line" management system. The three basic product lines would be spinal cord injury care, MS and outpatient services, and—the new one—acquired brain injury treatment.

"There are actually four," Ulicny clarifies, "if you count Medical/Surgical Care, the ICU, the whole acute care component, which is very much a part of what makes us unique." In fact, Shepherd Center is the only Spinal Cord Injury Model Center with med/surg and intensive care units, adding considerably to the hospital's stature and capabilities. Under the supervision of chief nursing executive Tracy Reed, RN, program director for medical/surgical services and intensive care, the 32-bed med-surg unit and eight-bed intensive care unit, located on the third floor of the Shepherd Building, enable Shepherd to care for patients before, during and after their rehabilitation.

In any event, Ulicny was quick to make his presence felt, and James Shepherd, for one, was applauding: "He's not bound by antiquated, traditional health care thinking; he's open to exploring new ways to deliver more efficient care less expensively while maintaining quality."

Of course, in addition to the best possible rehabilitative care, Shepherd's patients would continue to enjoy that incomparable range of "value-added" services

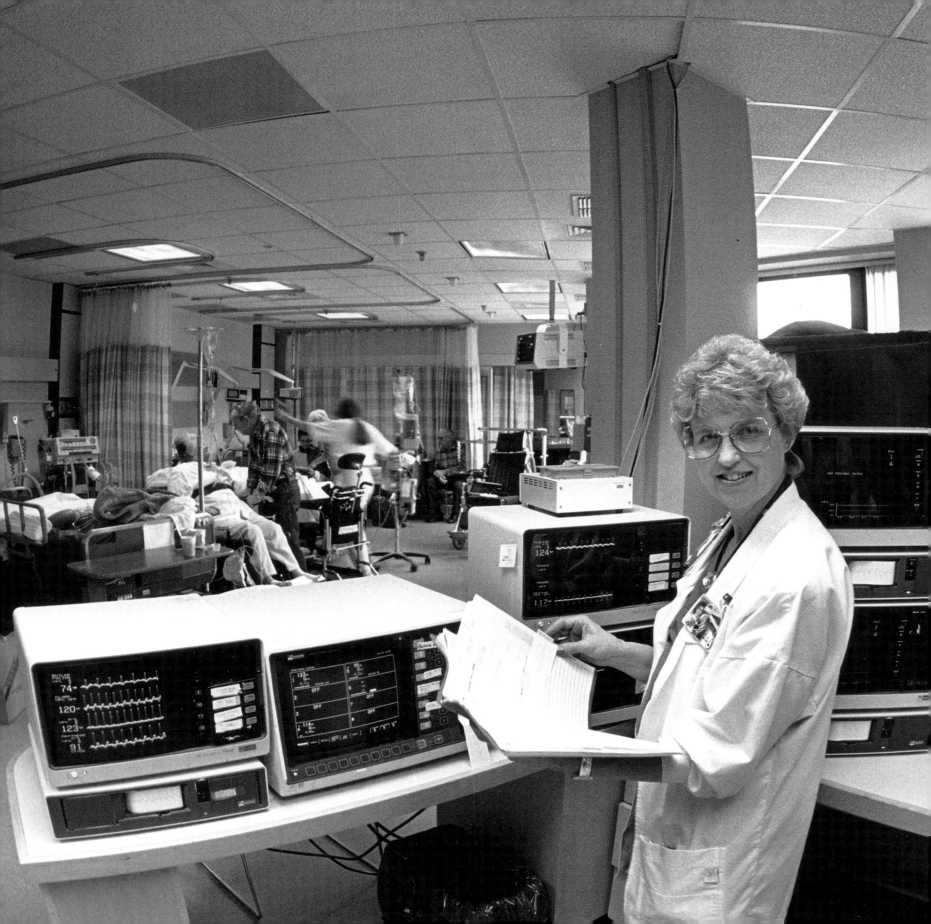

Vocational Services

When research data in the mid-80s revealed that a significant percentage of graduates were having difficulty returning to work, Shepherd was quick to respond. With the hiring of Darryle Craig, M.Ed., as the center's first employment specialist, Shepherd's employment program, as it was originally called, was officially up and running.

Fifteen years later, vocational services is one of the center's most visible—and most critical—programs. After all, in terms of the ultimate rehabilitation goal—i.e., reintegration into the life of the community—what could be more important than the return to work? Sally Atwell, manager since 1988, has guided the program's remarkable growth and development.

Though the vocational staff are experts in what Sally calls "traditional career counseling," the program's innovative approach reaches far outside Shepherd Center's walls. "For some patients," Sally explains, "the return to their old jobs is the motivating force behind their rehab. For such patients, and with their permission, we'll contact their employers, get a copy of the job description, and schedule a worksite visit if appropriate so that we can give that employer the information needed to bring this employee back to work."

Similarly, to bridge the gap between employer and employee, "We've made it our business to become experts on the government's programs and policies. Patients might fear an immediate loss of Social Security benefits if they return to work. On the other hand, employers might not be aware of the tax incentives involved in making their workplaces wheelchair accessible. So a lot of what we do is simply educating people."

Of the department's many creative solutions to the problem of matching the right person to the right job, one of the most successful has been its internship program, "Project Incubator." Initiated in 1992 with a major grant from the David, Helen and Marian Woodward Fund, the program matches job candidates with local employers to work a structured 90-day internship, with a stipend paid by Shepherd. "This is the perfect way to get our people out of the starting block," says Sally. "We set up the 90-day program with a contract that allays the employer's fears about future obligations to hire this person, about liability issues, and the like. At the end of the internship, all we ask is that if an appropriate position opens up our client be allowed to interview for it. At the very least, the intern gets a letter of recommendation and some valuable post-injury work experience."

The results of the program have been extremely rewarding, confirms Sally. "Of the people who have done internships, 68 percent have gone on to become employed."

Given the dramatic impact that vocational services has had on the lives of hundreds of former Shepherd patients, it seems especially fitting that Sally was named 1995 Counselor of the Year by the Georgia Rehabilitation Counseling Association. "This is the highest honor bestowed by GRCA," according to Mary Hollister-Cooke, the organization's president.

As for Sally, her personal reward comes, she says, "when the person you helped get a job ten years ago still keeps in touch. I asked this one guy we had worked with to come speak to a group for me, and he said, 'I'll do anything for you.' It's nice just to know that you've played a small part in a lot of people's rebuilding of their lives."

provided largely by the center's volunteer and donor community. That point was underscored by the opening of Shepherd's beautiful new chapel, funded by the Shepherd Center Auxiliary. With its elegant stained-glass window from Willett Studios in Philadelphia and its atmosphere of soothing serenity, the chapel "completes the wide range of services available through the pastoral care program," noted SSC chaplain Mike Moore.

At the same time, another value-added service received special recognition—with the unveiling along the first-floor corridor of the Marcus Building of the Walk of Fame. Created by Atlanta photographer Lynne Siler and still on view today, this inspiring exhibit features 20 photographic portraits of people in widely diverse occupations who found employment through Shepherd's vocational services program.

Sometimes the return to independence that culminates in finding challenging employment begins with regaining control of one's immediate environment. And that's where rehabilitative technology (or "assistive technology") comes in. Shepherd's effort to remain on the forefront of this rapidly advancing technology was given a boost in 1994 by a generous pledge of $25,000 from Bank South—funds that would go toward equipping a second assistive technology laboratory. The importance of this technology—a sip-and-puff mechanism, for example, that allows patients to access such basic services as the nurse call system or the telephone—cannot be exaggerated. "We've seen modifications such as these change a person's entire perspective," said Bill Nation, then the director of technology services.

Not that anybody at Shepherd was forgetting, but a summertime visit to the hospital by official mascot Blaze was a colorful reminder that the 1996 Paralympics would soon be imminent. Loosely based on Atlanta's own symbolic phoenix, Blaze perfectly embodied the spirit of the Paralympic athlete persevering in the face of adversity. "Blaze will be remembered as a great mascot," said Paralympics CEO Andy Fleming, "and his name certainly fits the definition of those who compete in these games." On August 16, a celebration at City Hall hosted by Mayor Bill Campbell and highlighted by the hoisting of the international Paralympic flag officially marked the beginning of the two-year countdown.

Meanwhile, corporate support for the games began to escalate with The Coca-Cola Company's announcement that it would be the 1996 Paralympics' first worldwide sponsor. Before the year was out, The Home Depot was also on board as a sponsor, with chairman and CEO Bernie Marcus announcing a commitment of $2 million in cash and another $2 million in in-kind products and services to APOC.

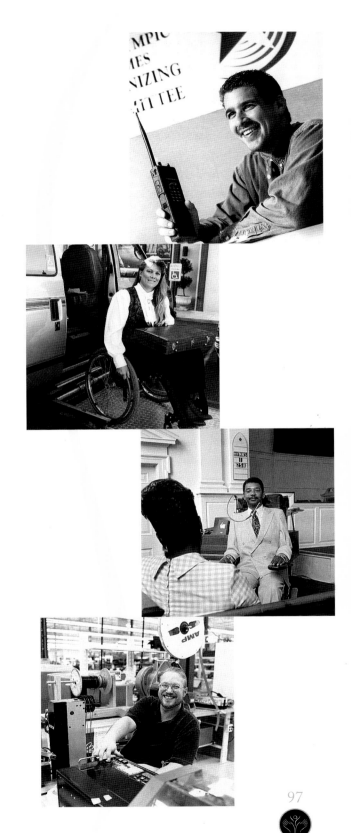

Hope Has a New Name

At age 20, Shepherd Spinal Center dropped its middle name. Reflecting the center's steady expansion into areas other than spinal cord injury—particularly with the fast-growing MS Center and the rapidly developing acquired brain injury (ABI) unit—it seemed appropriate to reshape the hospital's name in such a way as to suggest its ever-growing range of services. The new appellation: SHEPHERD CENTER—A Specialty Hospital. (Today, Shepherd defines itself as a "catastrophic care hospital.")

The name-change became official on May 4, at a special "Shepherd Center Day" celebration highlighted by a keynote address from James S. Brady, the former White House press secretary who sustained a brain injury from a gunshot wound during an assassination attempt upon President Ronald Reagan. A national advocate for gun control, Brady in 1995 was serving as vice chairman of the National Brain Injury Association. He concluded his remarks with a question—and an answer—that spoke to the heart of Shepherd's 20 years of service to the catastrophically injured: "What's the difference between a stumbling block and a stepping stone? It's all in the way you approach it."

The new name was ushered in along with the center's new blue and gold logo. In an era of rapid change in the health care field, the logo would serve as a reminder that Shepherd's basic mission would remain constant. "The hands represent Shepherd boosting people back out into the world again," said James Shepherd, "and the figure's arms are uplifted in hope and triumph, representing a celebration of independence and new abilities." Or, as Alana Shepherd observed, "The new logo shows the caring that sets us apart."

At the beginning of the hospital's third decade, it seemed clear that the pace of change would only accelerate, and Shepherd CEO Gary Ulicny was preparing his troops: "Shepherd Center will not remain static in the midst of health care turbulence; we are aggressively and proactively positioning ourselves to meet the future." But he, too, acknowledged that some things would not change: "In the midst of this transformation, we are maintaining the vital spirit of Shepherd: that we exist to bring people back to the highest possible level of independence and that we go the extra mile to make that happen."

As a final highlight to this special anniversary year, Shepherd Center received five memorable gifts from particularly generous benefactors.

- Paul Bowen, who for many years had been one of the center's most faithful volunteers—and one of the originators of the Patient Feeding Program—donated the accumulated cash value of a life insurance policy in memory of his wife.

- Mildred and Norman Elsas, also longtime supporters, named Shepherd as one of the institutions to benefit from the charitable remainder annuity trust created by their estate.

- Although unaware of it until the will was read, Shepherd was also named as a major beneficiary of the estate of Marion Troy Davis, who quietly bequeathed to the center more than a half-million dollars.

- Another heartwarming surprise was provided by the will of Mabel Shropshire, who made Shepherd the primary beneficiary of her estate. The more than $2 million bequest was the second-largest single gift in Shepherd's history.

- And finally, Cile and Charlie Davidson and their children, great admirers of the Shepherd family and Shepherd Center, donated a 42 percent interest in 162 acres of undeveloped land in DeKalb County—one of the largest-ever real estate gifts to Shepherd Center.

Fittingly, the year came to a close with a special tribute: James Shepherd and Shepherd Center were honored as recipients of the 1995 National Rehabilitation Week John Heinz Memorial Award—one of the most prestigious in the field of rehabilitation medicine. Tom Pugh of Allied Services, a provider of rehabilitation services and sponsor of National Rehabilitation Week, made the presentation: "Shepherd Center is committed to awareness advocacy, employment of people with disabilities, clinical research, and rehabilitation education, and it reflects James Shepherd's personal desire to positively impact the quality of life for people with disabilities."

Nobody could be affiliated with Shepherd without feeling compelled to give something back. Great credit goes to Alana and James for instilling that spirit here. A place like this doesn't happen unless people love what they're doing and feel passionately committed to it.

—Curtis Rodgers
Coordinator, Peer Support

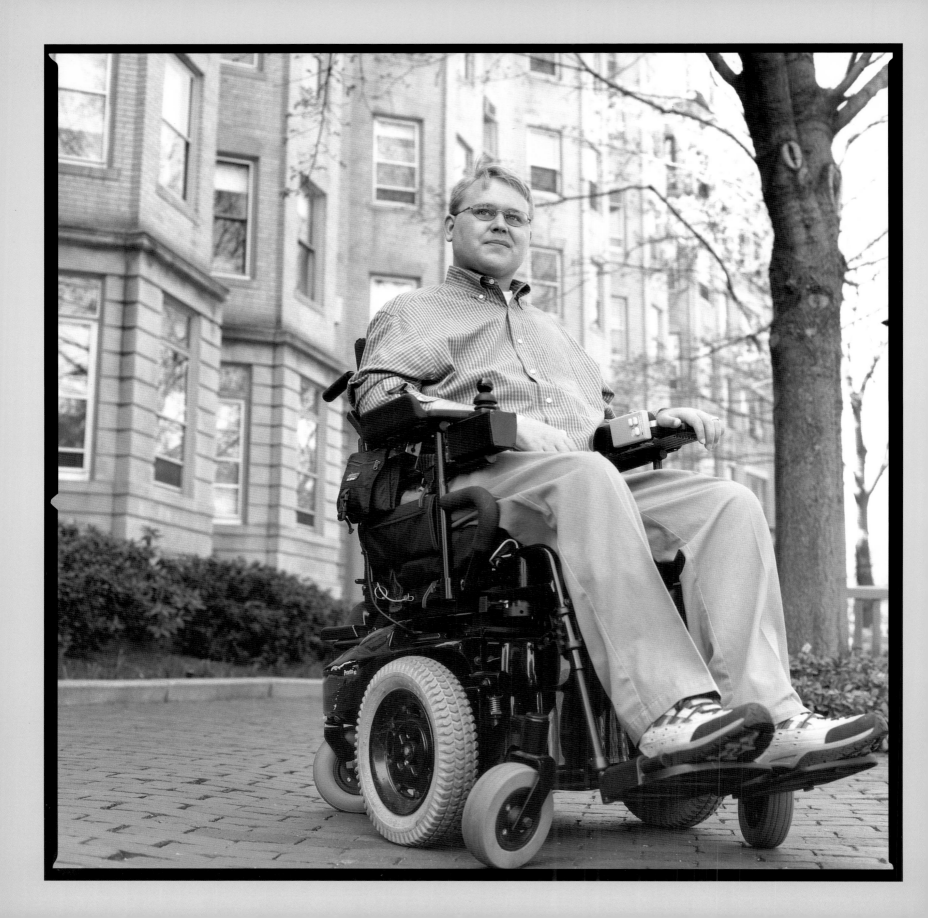

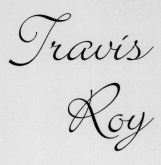

Travis Roy

"knew something was wrong, and paralysis did cross my mind," says Travis Roy, recalling the head-first collision that broke his neck just 11 seconds into his first college hockey game. His parents, sister, and girlfriend were in the stands that night to cheer Travis on. They saw him hit the boards, fall, and not get up. In the blink of an eye, this highly recruited hockey star had a journey unfolding in front of him that couldn't have been more different from the one he'd always envisioned.

For three and a half months, Travis remained in a Boston hospital, breathing through a ventilator and battling pneumonia, infections, a pressure sore and depression. He got out of bed only twice during the entire stay.

His mother visited Shepherd, and on the strength of her recommendation, Travis decided to make the long trip to Atlanta. The day after he arrived, he was in a wheelchair for the first time and his rehabilitation was underway.

Also underway was a veritable tidal wave of media attention, and, for Travis, an unlooked for new role as celebrity spokesperson for the spinal cord injured. Good Morning America, The Today Show, CNN, network news programs, and countless newspapers reported on Travis's accident, his therapy, his progress, his plans for the future.

Travis weathered the storm with fortitude and grace, answering every question — even the most personal and insensitive ones — with honesty and quiet candor. In the process, he brought attention to the phenomenon of spinal cord injury like few people ever had before. "This isn't what I wanted to be known for," said Travis at the time. "I dreamed of being famous for other reasons. But I've been put in a position where I might be able to do some good."

Travis returned to Boston University and graduated in four years, a communications major and proud member of the class of 2000. The full course load at BU didn't quite deplete Travis's energy, however. During the year after his accident, he wrote a book about the experience, Eleven Seconds, which was published by Warner Books in 1997. "It sold pretty well," he says. "I think Warner was pleased." What's more, an independent filmmaker in Boston bought the rights to the story and plans to make a feature film. "But that's a slower process," says Travis, "and it's still in development."

Also while still a student Travis created the Travis Roy Foundation. "We raise money through fundraisers like golf tournaments, regattas, and the like, and also solicit corporate donations," Travis explains. "Half of the proceeds go to spinal cord research, and the other half goes to individual grants to help people purchase adaptive equipment."

Since leaving Shepherd, Travis says he has stayed "very busy and very healthy," and he's deeply appreciative of the help he got at Shepherd.

"Shepherd was a wonderful place for me," he says. "The people there really turned my attitude around. They got me to see bright light again."

To this day he gets calls from people who have just been spinal cord injured and who remember his story. "They want to know what to do," Travis says, "and the first thing I say is, 'Can you get to Shepherd?'"

(Thanks to Julie Kinzel's profile of Travis, "The Whole World Watching," Spinal Column, Summer 1996, pp. 18-19.)

> "Shepherd was a wonderful place for me. The people there really turned my attitude around. They got me to see bright light again."

And then 1996 brought the Paralympic Games to Atlanta, the unqualified success of which was in no small part attributable to the dedication of the entire Shepherd Center community.

"It was so much like the early days of the Auxiliary," remembers Sara Chapman, who served as chairman of the Volunteer Advisory Committee. "We were just trying to stay one step ahead of the athletes, of the events. We were setting up flags, making sure the medals were ready, doing everything. It was a small staff and a huge volunteer force, and the volunteers did everything, except maybe for driving Vice President Al Gore around." Sara's committee eventually would recruit close to 10,000 volunteers, mostly from local corporations, with volunteers from each company taking charge of a particular venue.

Of course, those corporate volunteers were given the time off to help with the Paralympic effort. Not so with Shepherd folks. As Montez Howard recalls, "We all really had two or three jobs that year. Unlike the corporate people who would get the day off, we worked all day here at Shepherd, then worked at the Paralympics at night. But we loved it; it was a really great opportunity. And it makes me realize how great our staff is, in its extraordinary energy level and creativity."

As APOC president and CEO Andy Fleming declared upon the games' arrival: "If it hadn't been for Shepherd Center's involvement, the Paralympic Games wouldn't be here today."

"That's why a whole new category was created for us," explains Mark Johnson. "Founding Sponsor. There was only one. We gave time, energy, advocacy, but since we didn't have a lot of money to give, we didn't qualify as a sponsor in the traditional sense. We made it happen, though."

The final statistics confirm the size of the undertaking. The Games brought to Atlanta 3,310 athletes from 104 nations, who participated in 17 different sports over 10 days of competition. And by the way, the Paralympians established 268 new world records in Atlanta.

Capping its five years of work in capturing and then preparing for the Paralympics, during the actual 10-day event Shepherd provided more than 120 medical and sports volunteers to organize, judge, and support the competition. At the same time, other staffers were busy organizing sports demonstrations, art shows, educational sessions, receptions, and tours. In addition, the center provided uniforms for those 10,000 volunteers Sara Chapman's committee recruited and created the Games' official countdown sign.

When it was all over, nobody doubted that the monumental effort had been well worthwhile—not only because of the Games' overwhelming success but also because of their legacy for the future. For one thing, as Mark Johnson points out, "Nobody will have to fight this fight again. From now on, the Olympic host city

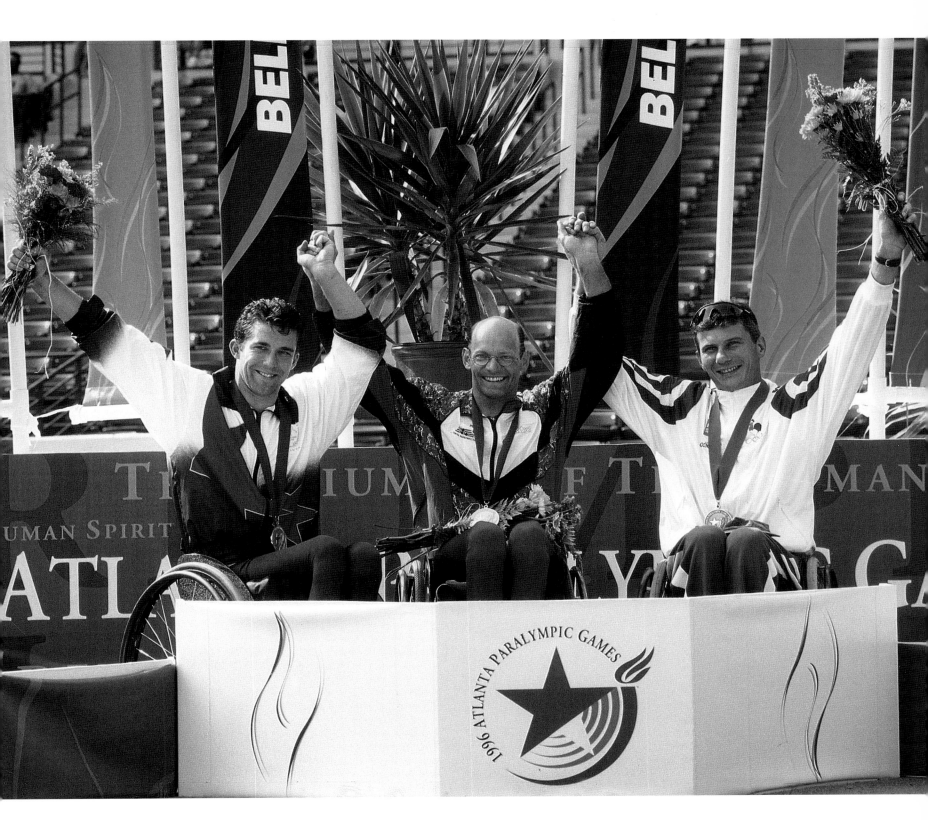

automatically hosts the Paralympics." Another lasting benefit—for Atlanta and all future Paralympic site cities—would be a permanently heightened consciousness on the issue of accessibility. However, as Andy Fleming pointed out, accessibility is just the beginning: "The real legacy of these Games is not found in infrastructure, but in humanity."

Fleming's view was substantiated by the remarkable success of the Third Paralympic Congress, which ran concurrently with the Games. Close to one thousand conferees from more than 50 nations came together to address human rights, economic opportunity, and access to sports for people with disabilities. Of course, Shepherd was well represented, with staffers Ann Temkin, Jim Krause, Ginny Posid, Paula Maiberger, Stacy Green, Mike Hufstetler and Pat Driscoll presenting at the various symposia. Meanwhile, Mark Johnson and Sally Atwell led two of the all-important "consensus" sessions—Mark's on human rights and Sally's on employment of people with disabilities.

Montez Howard, for one, remembers the Congress as the defining moment of the Paralympic experience: "It was the first time that so many people involved in disability activism throughout the nation and world came together in one room. To be there listening to those people was a special time for me."

(In fact, thanks to the efforts of those many people, before the arrival of the 2000 Olympics the U.S. Congress had amended the Olympic and Amateur Sports Act with a number of provisions on behalf of disabled athletes. For example, the United States Olympic Committee would henceforth be recognized as the National Paralympic Committee for the U.S., and athletes with disabilities would be considered "amateur athletes" under the Act, entitled to the same rights and opportunities granted to all amateur athletes.)

Not to be forgotten in the whirlwind leading up to the Paralympics, on July 4 the Wheelchair Division of the Peachtree Road Race celebrated its 15th anniversary. Under the official sponsorship of Shepherd Center since 1984, the event had by 1996 grown to become the largest wheelchair 10K race in the country. "Another great event," says Alana Shepherd, "and great for our patients. They are out there watching, and some of them determine that one day they'll be among the ones participating. That's the real reason for it; that's what makes it so important."

Therapeutic Recreation

Shepherd Center's original "value added" program, therapeutic recreation (TR) probably demonstrates Shepherd's commitment to the total rehabilitation of its patients like no other single program. Always a part of Dr. David Apple's and James Shepherd's vision of what spinal cord rehabilitation must encompass, the program was officially inaugurated in January, 1979, with the hiring of Barb Leidheiser (now Trader), as Shepherd Center's first therapeutic recreation specialist.

"I give Barb all the credit in the world," says Mike Hufstetler, who joined Barb's staff in 1987 as an outdoor specialist. "She had the desire and the ability to create this department, and she did it."

Now Mike directs the department, one of Shepherd's largest and most visible. "We have inpatient therapists," explains Mike, "who meet with each patient, determine his or her interests, do an assessment, and develop a plan. When appropriate, our therapists then place the patients under one or more of our five specialists—outdoor, art, sports, aquatic, and horticulture. That's what sets our TR department apart. We have so much to offer our patients that we can really make an impact."

Like other departments throughout the hospital, therapeutic recreation is coping with the effects of managed care—particularly the dramatically shortened length of stay for the typical inpatient. "The problem is," says Mike, "that patients are no longer here long enough to build up the strength and stamina for many of the recreational activities we are able to offer. Of course we still do a lot of things, but we move at a slower pace to accommodate the patients' intensified and tightened schedule of daily activities."

Also, typical of Shepherd's philosophy of the "continuum of care," therapeutic recreation continues to work with patients after they leave the hospital. "We're always looking for new ways to deliver our services to patients after they've left the hospital," says Mike, "whether by providing them with instructional videos that they can work with at home or by encouraging them to return and participate on one of our sports teams."

Widely recognized for its development of the Wheelchair Division of the Peachtree Road Race into a world-class event, Shepherd's TR department is winning nationwide acclaim on other fronts as well. Mike is especially proud of the annual Adventure Skills Workshop, where approximately fifty wheelchair campers from across the country—including former and current Shepherd patients—gather at a campground in Alabama for a long weekend of outdoor activities: water skiing, canoeing, wave running, kayaking, scuba diving, trailriding on ATVs, skeet shooting, fishing, horseback riding, and more. "It's the largest and most successful camp of its kind," says Mike, "and it has brought us lots of attention.

Mike also points out the success of the inaugural performing arts festival in 1999, coordinated by Pam McClure, the department's art specialist. "In another year or two," he says, "we expect that event to rise to the level of the Wheelchair Division of the Peachtree Road Race and the Adventure Skills Workshop."

Which should surprise no one. "As we identify worthwhile new programs," says Mike, "I think we'll find a way to make them happen. That's always been the way here at Shepherd."

Inside Shepherd's walls, the big story of 1996 was the dedication of the Virginia C. Crawford Research Institute. Thanks to one of the largest individual gifts ever made to Shepherd, the Institute would bolster the center's critical—and groundbreaking—research effort, long a hallmark of Shepherd's excellence. "Virginia's gift provides the foundation that will allow us to expand our clinical research program and share the results with people affected by catastrophic injuries and illnesses worldwide," as Alana gratefully acknowledged.

The gift was yet another remarkable contribution by one of the center's most loyal and notable benefactors. Mrs. Crawford served as vice president of Shepherd's board of directors for its first 20 years, stepping down in 1995 to become the center's first honorary director. Her many generous donations over the years include a major gift for the Virginia C. Crawford Nutrition Center in 1985 and another one to the capital campaign for the construction of The Billi Marcus Building. A life member of the Auxiliary, Mrs. Crawford was named Shepherd's Angel of the Year in 1986 and Honorary Chairman of the first Legendary Party in 1989.

Among those most appreciative of Mrs. Crawford's gift was Michael L. Jones, Ph.D., appointed in 1996 as Shepherd's new research director. Arriving from North Carolina State University, where he had served as director of the Center for Universal Design, Mike had worked as a research coordinator as well as an investigator in numerous rehabilitation-related research studies. As research director at Shepherd, Mike assumed responsibility for developing new research projects, monitoring ongoing projects, and soliciting research grants from the scientific community.

Mike no doubt also appreciated the fact that Shepherd Center's designation as a Model Center had just been renewed for the fifth time by the National Institute on Disability and Rehabilitation Research. And again, the special designation came with a five-year, $1.9 million grant to initiate and participate in research related to spinal cord injury. Shepherd remained the only Model Center in Georgia, one of only two in the Southeast, and one of but 17 in the entire country.

Meanwhile, the MS Center at Shepherd was announcing an exciting research venture of its own: the Shepherd/Harvard MS Research Initiative. Two pioneering MS researchers from Harvard—Drs. David A. Hafler and Howard L. Weiner—were affiliating with Shepherd to collaborate with the MS Center medical staff.

The initiative was spearheaded by Atlanta's Bill Fowler, a board member of both Shepherd Center and the Georgia Chapter of the National Multiple Sclerosis Society—and also an MS patient. When Bill discovered he had MS, he quickly sought out Dr. Hafler, the renowned MS expert at Harvard Medical

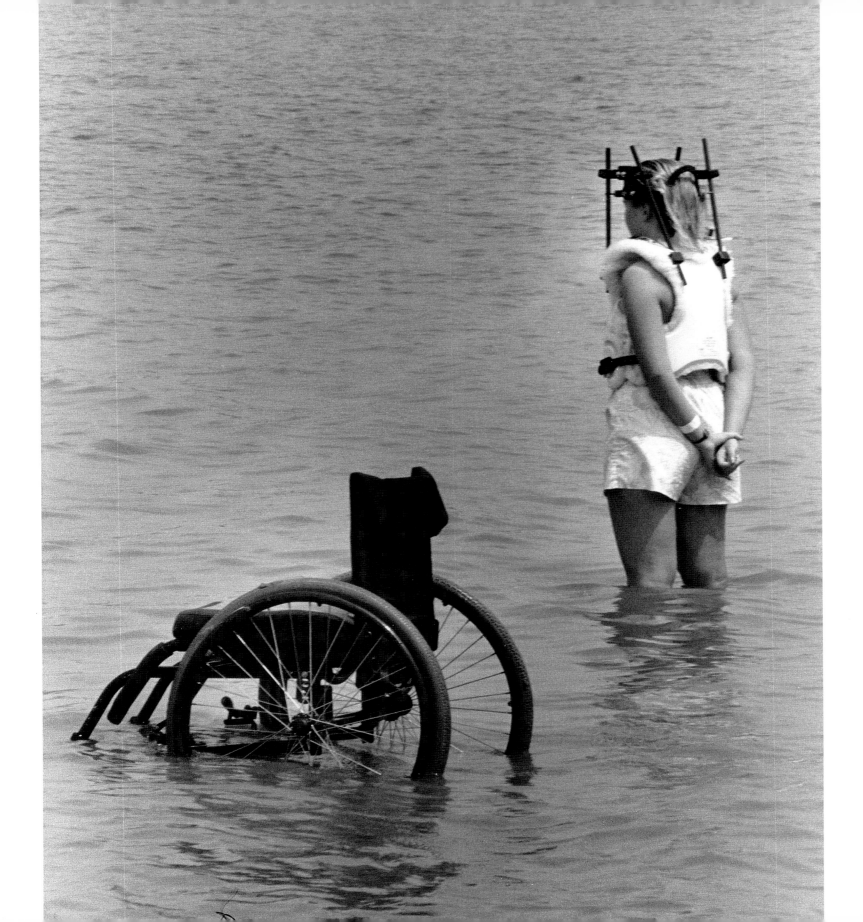

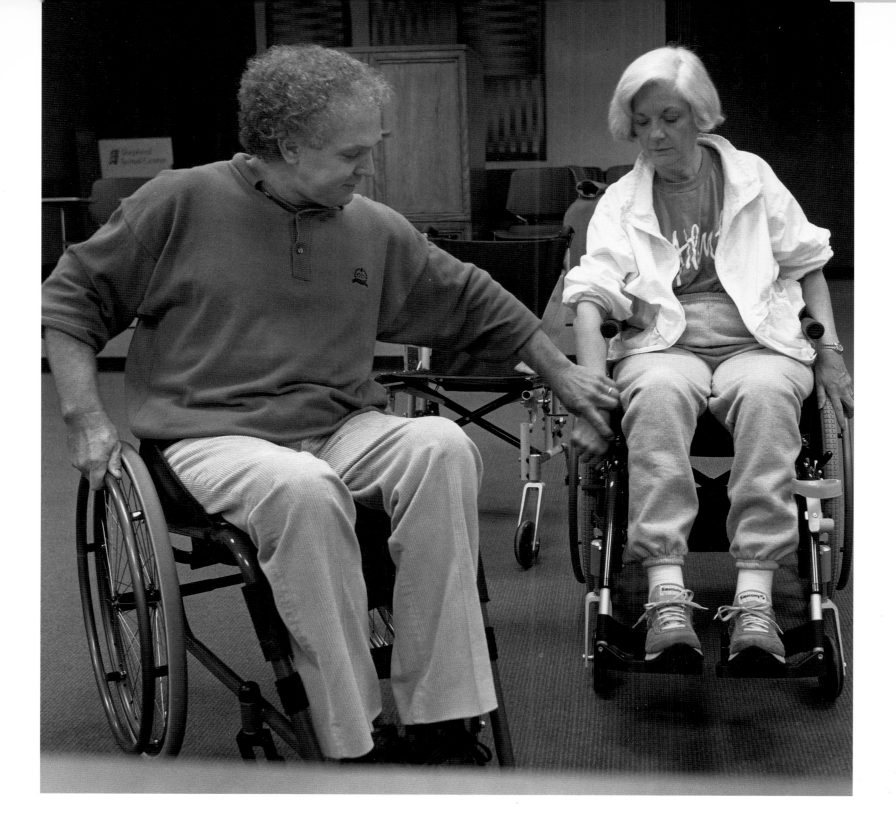

School. When he subsequently needed a physician in Atlanta to administer Dr. Hafler's prescribed treatment, Bill came to Dr. William Stuart at Shepherd. By bringing the two doctors together, Bill saw a chance to realize his dream—"to have Harvard's leading-edge multiple sclerosis research findings available for all the people of Georgia."

The relationship is still going strong and it's been very successful in a number of ways. Shepherd has been involved in some good collaborative research and developed strong relationships with other people on the cutting edge of medical science. It has also given Shepherd rapid credibility in the research arena—which is not easy to achieve.

Even before the arrival of the Harvard researchers, though, Shepherd was already being selected by Berlex Laboratories as one of thirty MS centers nationally to clinically test the drug Betaseron. This would be the first major clinical drug trial since the 1960s available to people in the Southeast. With Betaseron already having proved effective in the treatment of relapsing-remitting MS, the new three-year study would test the drug against secondary progressive MS, defined as a history of relapses and remissions followed by progressive deterioration for at least six months. The MS Center at Shepherd was the only test site selected in Georgia. For our overall research effort, that was very validating.

Finally, from Shepherd's exemplary community of supporters and volunteers, 1996 brought two very welcome stories—one of deep generosity and the other of well-deserved recognition.

First, it was learned that Herbert I. Gordy and his wife, Lilla, had bequeathed more than $3 million to the hospital. Gordy was the owner of Gordy Tire Co. and a longtime friend and business associate of Harold Shepherd. "When we started the center in 1975," recalled Harold, "he gave us a generous donation, but he told me just prior to his death that he never thought he'd given us enough." Thus the bequest.

And second, having given untold time and energy to Shepherd ever since her college days 17 years earlier, board member Sara Chapman was a recipient of the 11-Alive Community Service Awards from WXIA-TV. Sara was honored for her many years of service to the center (where she has been president of the Auxiliary, co-chairman of the Junior Committee, advisory board member, and member of the board of directors, among many other endeavors) as well as for her role as chairman of the Paralympics Volunteer Advisory Committee.

Alana has been such an inspiration, such an incredible mentor. She'd say, "Come on, Sara, we're gonna make this happen. The worst they can say is no. Let's go for it."

—Sara Chapman
Member, Board of Directors

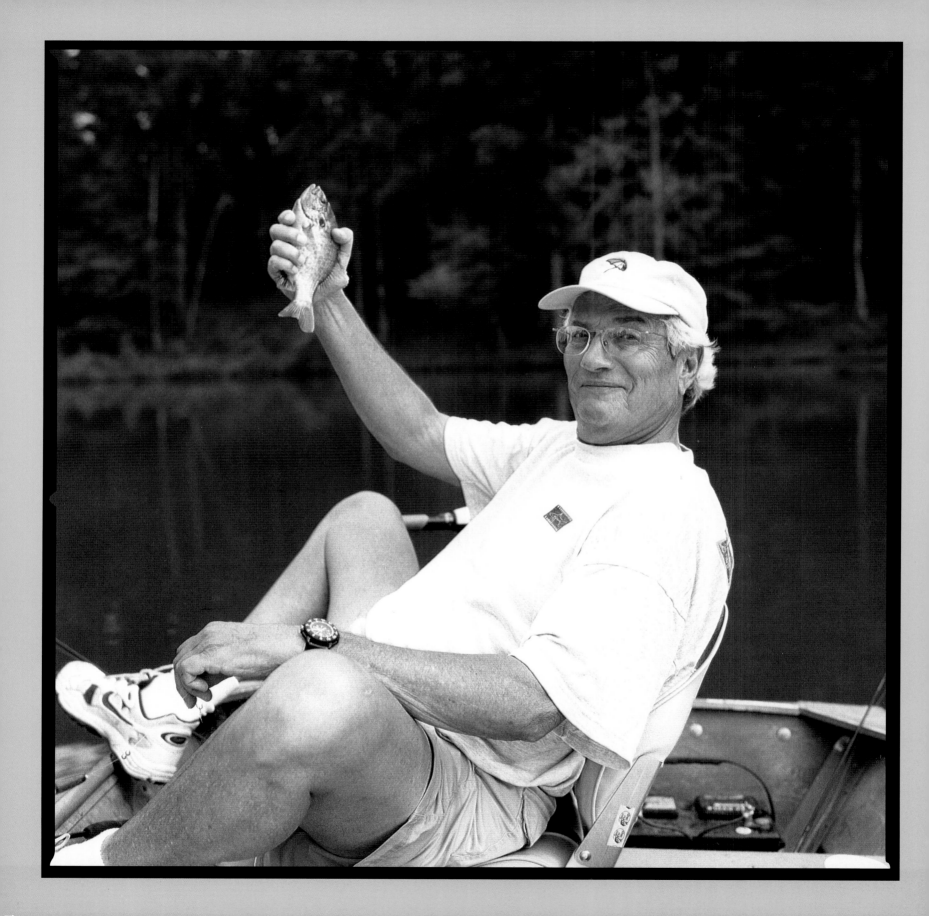

When C. L Straughn reached for a coffee cup one morning and found himself unable to pick it up, he went straight to his doctor.

"They put me in the hospital, I got better, I came home, and then my legs gave out on me. I went back to the hospital and I stayed there about a year that time." This was in 1995, which C. L. remembers because he got out of the hospital just as the 1996 Olympics were coming to Atlanta.

"All kinds of things started happening to me," C. L. continues. "My blood pressure was high, and since kidney problems cause high blood pressure, they were treating me for kidney disease. Finally they diagnosed me as having Guillain Barré Syndrome. (Guillain Barré Syndrome is an unpredictable, inflammatory disorder of the nerves outside the brain and spinal cord that can cause weakness or paralysis in the legs, arms, breathing muscles and face.)

Once he was diagnosed, C. L. credits Shepherd Center for reversing the course of the disease. "In the first place," he says, "I had been lying in Piedmont Hospital on a ventilator for six months, and Shepherd got me off of it. If they hadn't got me off that ventilator, I guess I'd've died."

Over the course of 90 days as an inpatient and another five months as an outpatient, C. L.'s recovery progressed steadily. "The people at Shepherd were wonderful," he says. "They had to get me walking all over again. I went from a wheelchair, to a walker, to crutches, to a cane, and then to nothing."

Today his recovery is almost complete: "I'm doing quite well," he says. "My feet haven't come back 100 percent — there's still some numbness in them — but I still walk and play golf and bird hunt — pretty much everything I've ever done."

Including resume his career as a real estate developer. The disease cost him two years, and he readily admits that he was fortunate to be able to afford it. "I was lucky to have had some money in the bank and everything paid for and no debt; otherwise, I don't know. Not working for two years, you know, will put most people in the poorhouse." Now, C. L. says, he's working harder than ever before.

C. L. is quick to include his family in his embrace of gratitude. "My wife was a life saver. She looked after me like nobody in the world. Why, for two years I couldn't drive a car. Sometimes I wonder if the shoe was on the other foot would I have been able to handle it as well as she did. My two daughters were also very supportive. I had a great family behind me."

Except for his feet, C. L. describes himself as "in perfect health," and he expects that last symptom to disappear. "They say that the nerves regenerate themselves at a rate of an inch a month. So that's about five years down to the tip of your toes. I'm actually ahead of schedule, and they tell me the feeling will come back."

His feeling for Shepherd never diminished. "If ever there was a saint on this earth, it's Alana Shepherd. There was not a single day that I was in that hospital that she didn't come visit me, and encourage me.

"I have a big place in my heart for Shepherd Center," he declares. "I really feel like Alana and that hospital saved my life."

C. L. Straughn

"I had been lying in Piedmont Hospital on a ventilator for six months, and Shepherd got me off of it. If they hadn't got me off that ventilator, I guess I'd've died."

Opposite: Shepherd
Pathways on Clairmont
Road

With the hiring of Gary Ulicny in 1994, and with Gary's hiring of Mike Jones in 1996, Shepherd Center was strategically positioning itself to pursue its mission within the dramatically reconfigured medical arena known as managed care.

Though felt everywhere, the heavy constraints of managed care were most strikingly visible in the mandated reduced length of inpatient care, with the average length of stay dropping from 72 days to 42. Or, as Gary describes the evolving scenario, "We're serving more patients, but doing it in about half the time and getting paid less than half of what we used to. So the question we face is how to cut costs, stay competitive, and continue to provide quality care." How indeed? Throughout the end of the decade and on into the 21st century, the course of Shepherd's growth and development would be directed by its effort to address this question.

One immediate answer was the hiring of Mitch Fillhaber in the position of vice president of marketing/managed care. A 20-year veteran in the health care/marketing arena, Mitch's job would be to make sure Shepherd remained the provider of choice for treatment of catastrophic injuries. Today Mitch negotiates managed care contracts with more than 30 insurance companies, the companies that often make the decisions as to where the catastrophically injured should be hospitalized. The image that Shepherd presents to potential managed care partners—and to the world—is in the hands of Mitch and his capable marketing/public relations staff.

"But more generally," says Gary Ulicny, "our response to managed care lies in our research program." For example, the branch of research that Mike Jones refers to as "health services delivery" deals directly with managed care issues. "We used to use the 'inoculation model,'" explains Mike, "where we 'inoculate' patients against anything that might happen to them post discharge. But now we simply don't have time to do that, so we search for alternative methods."

Thus such innovations as the day hospital program, designed to continue in-depth rehabilitation after the termination of the maximum allowable in-hospital stay. Or Shepherd's cutting-edge research into telemedicine, which combines telephone lines and video technology to allow doctors and clinicians to "visit" patients—see them on the video screen and monitor their rehabilitation—after they have returned home. "A classic example of services delivery," says Mike.

Or, as of August 1997, Shepherd Pathways, Shepherd's newly purchased facility at 1942 Clairmont Road in DeKalb County. Formerly the home of Restore Rehabilitation Group, Shepherd saw the acquisition of the property as a way to expand its ABI program and better manage the full recovery of its patients with brain injuries. Created for patients who have completed the acute phase of

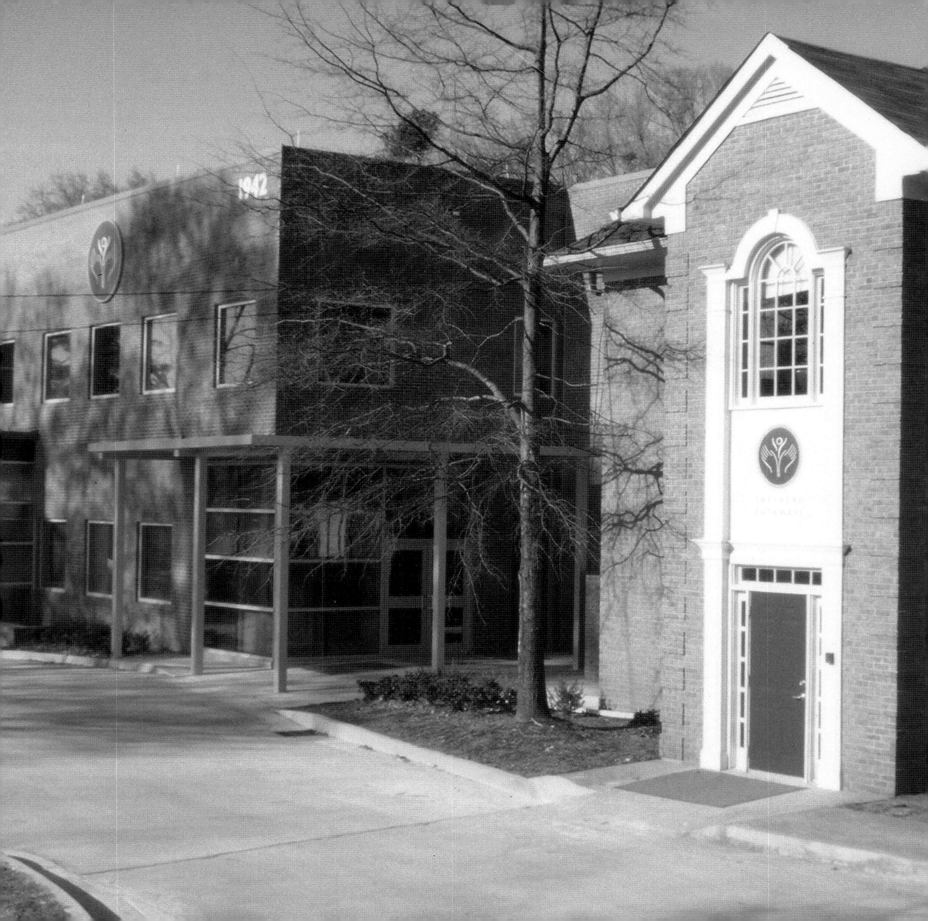

their treatment but still require comprehensive rehabilitation services, Shepherd Pathways constituted a "step down" into community-based outpatient services. "With Shepherd Pathways," said Dr. Donald Leslie, medical director of the ABI program, "we are able to offer more comprehensive services at competitive pricing, enhancing our position as the largest ABI rehabilitation provider in the state."

As Mike Jones points out, clinical research has long been another critical component of the total research effort, but particularly with the inception of the Crawford Research Institute, this was an area in which Shepherd's visibility seemed to skyrocket. "In terms of our excellence in clinical services," Mike explains, "in sheer numbers of patients served, and in expertise to serve those patients, there's no other place like Shepherd in the country—or the world. And what's happened is that the people in the government agencies in charge of funding research have begun to sit up and take notice."

In Shepherd's urology department, for example, a number of groundbreaking clinical trials were already underway as Mike settled into his role as research director. According to Shepherd urologist Dr. Wylly Killorin, Jr., the hospital was conducting a test of the effectiveness of the drug Terazosin in the treatment of bladder obstruction. "Preliminary results look favorable," said Dr. Killorin—no doubt to the delight of the 30 Shepherd patients fortunate enough to be enrolled in the trial. In addition, Shepherd was the trial site for collagen urethral implantation, a procedure in which collagen is injected into tissues around the urethra to add "bulk," thus allowing it to close more tightly and prevent leakage. Performed on an outpatient basis, this procedure was proving effective in 80 percent of trial patients.

Meanwhile, after having been involved with the clinical trial of Betaseron, the MS Center at Shepherd was selected to participate in the study of Copaxone, a synthetic form of myelin, the fatty substance that protects nerve fibers in the brain and spinal cord. Thanks to the success of these and other developing MS drug therapies, patients' attitudes were changing for the better. Some of our therapies began to show modifying potential, and this is what patients were coming to us for. They began to get the sense that at least somebody was trying to help them, rather than the traditional response—i.e., go home, there's nothing to be done.

Before the end of the year came one last remarkable piece of research-related news. The National Institute on Disability and Rehabilitation Research, which 15 years earlier had designated Shepherd a "Model Center" in spinal cord injury and had since that time continually renewed it generous research grant, now designated Shepherd a "Model Center" for the treatment of brain injury as well. In collaboration with Emory University Hospital, Shepherd Center was awarded a $1.38 million grant to fund the Georgia Model Brain Injury System (GAMBIS).

"It's a wonderful irony," says Dr. Donald Leslie, medical director of the brain injury unit, "because frankly, I was initially reluctant to bring brain injury here. We had such a marvelous spinal cord program, one of the best anywhere, and brain injury is very different, very difficult and challenging. But it made sense, given the number of dual-diagnosis patients (patients with spinal cord and brain injury) we had already treated, and the transition was quite smooth. Still, the fact that after only two years we were selected as a model brain injury program is a great tribute to what we've accomplished. And we are one of very few—a very small handful—of hospitals in the country that have Model programs in both spinal cord injury and brain injury."

The federal government was abetting Shepherd's mission in a less direct way as well—or trying to. In June of 1997, then-House Speaker Newt Gingrich—with no little prodding from Shepherd's advocacy specialist Mark Johnson—introduced HR 2020, the Medicaid Community Attendant Services Act (CASA), which, in terms of disability rights, was considered the most important piece of legislation since the Americans with Disabilities Act (ADA). Potentially a tremendous advance in a battle Shepherd Center had been fighting for more than five years, the bill would allow Medicaid patients eligible for nursing home or other institutional services to choose in-home attendant care instead. (Unfortunately, CASA never made it out of the House. But, according to Mark, a new version, Medicaid Community Attendant Services and Support Act [MiCASSA] is currently pending.)

And speaking of the ADA, the summer of 1997 also marked the inauguration of Initiative 2000, a three-year celebration of the passing of that landmark legislation that would culminate with a ten-year anniversary festival in July 2000. The event would be highlighted by a nationwide torch relay, the final stop of which would be New York City on August 7. Fittingly, the relay would come to Atlanta and Shepherd Center, on July 20—21.

This year also brought special recognition to Dr. David Apple, Shepherd's founding medical director. The American Spinal Injury Association (ASIA), the premier organization for spinal cord injury physicians, awarded Dr. Apple its Lifetime Achievement Award, its ultimate accolade.

My fifteen years here have been the best time of my life. It's an incredible place.

—Dr. Donald P. Leslie
Associate Medical Director
and Medical Director,
Outpatient Services
and ABI Program

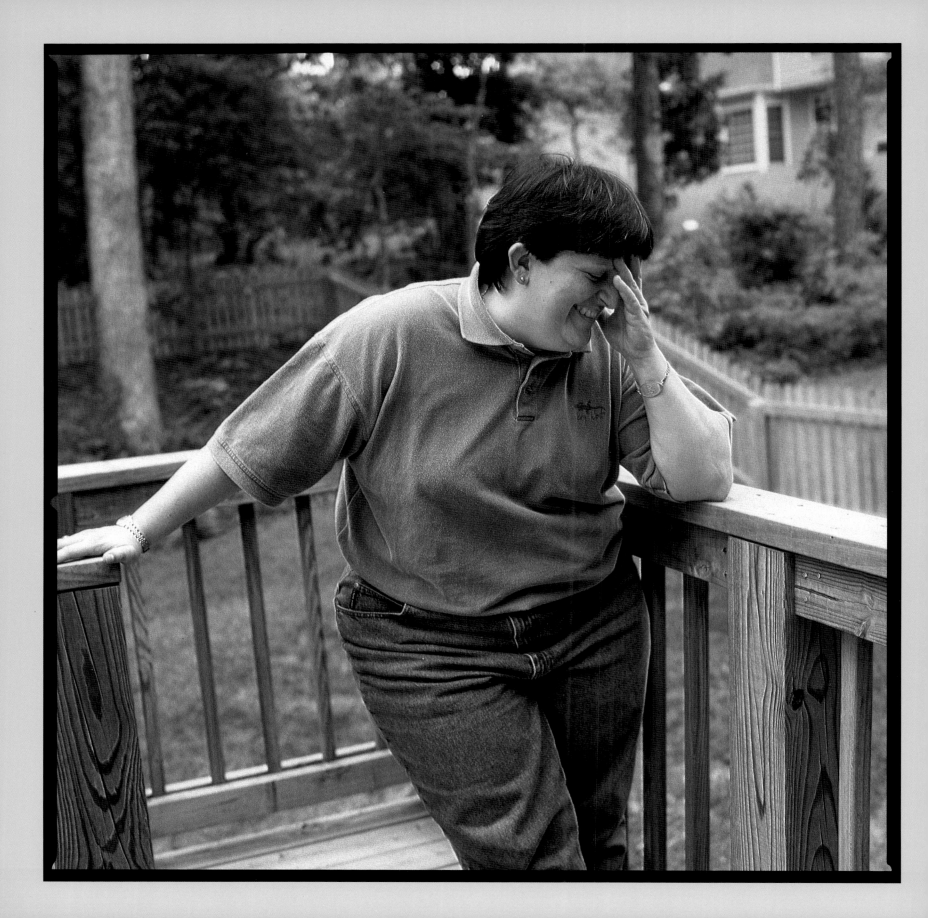

*P*at Cocciolone was in her tenth year as an Atlanta police officer — a job she loved dearly — when she was shot while responding to a domestic call in October 1997. Her fellow officer, John Sowa was killed in the assault. Pat's hip was shattered by one bullet; another entered her brain two inches above her left temple and exited behind her ear.

"That shot," she would later write in Spinal Column (Summer 1998), "changed my life."

Pat was rushed to Grady Hospital, where she underwent emergency surgery to remove bone fragments from her brain and to repair her shattered hip. Five weeks later, still unable to walk or talk, she was transferred to Shepherd.

"I still didn't feel well," Pat wrote. "As a matter of fact, I felt like I was about to throw up most of the time. I recognized my best friend, Carole Henry, and my two brothers right away, but it took a long time for me to recognize any of my fellow officers, and I still didn't know what had happened."

Pat was placed under the care of Dr. Donald Leslie, medical director of Shepherd's acquired brain injury program, whose team worked with Pat on cognition, comprehension, and walking. In addition to the severe pain from the hip injury, Pat suffered from acute dizziness and blindness in both eyes in the right portion of her field of vision. Even worse, she had lost the ability to express her self verbally and to understand language and the written word.

Her therapy has been difficult and demanding, just as her progress has been steady and encouraging. "I knew I was going to be okay the first day I walked," wrote Pat. "People were holding onto me and helping me, but I still did it. I was so happy."

One of her therapies allowed Pat to return to a beloved hobby, playing the acoustic guitar. "Working with familiar sounds and her favorite folk songs," reported Shepherd's music specialist Eric Manolson, "Pat's able to look at sheet music and play the right chords, even though she can't yet read the words."

Today, however, reading has taken precedence over guitar playing. According to Carole Williams, Pat's attendant, now that she has begun to read again, she is putting all her energy into that. And the reading homework that constitutes her therapy is piling up.

Carole adds that Pat's speaking has progressed greatly, and that her spirits are really good, "though at times she still gets a little aggravated that all this has happened."

Pat stays busy at the job of getting well. She drives herself to Shepherd, where she remains in Dr. Leslie's care, as well as to other therapists around the city. And she's playing an active role with the Brain and Spinal Injury Trust Fund Authority. Governor Barnes appointed her to the authority for a two-year term, and she's totally involved in this new endeavor.

In Pat's own words: "The best thing about getting well is knowing that I'm going to be okay — no, more than okay."

(Thanks to Michele Upchurch, who contributed to Pat's profile of herself, "The Shot That Changed My Life," Spinal Column, Summer 1998, pp. 8-10.)

Patricia Cocciolone

"I knew I was going to be okay the first day I walked. People were holding onto me and helping me, but I still did it. I was so happy."

Shepherd Center's mission to create "a complete continuum of care" for the spinal cord injured would not languish while politicians in Washington debated the merits of independent care. With a new initiative, ShepherdCare, Shepherd joined forces with the Georgia Department of Medical Assistance to enhance the health care services of Medicaid recipients with disabilities who have been accepted into the state's Medicaid Independent Care Waiver Program. Under the direction of Tammy King, ShepherdCare provides a rehabilitation nurse/case manager to make sure that the appropriate services are being rendered and that the Medicaid dollars are put to the best possible use.

Typical of Shepherd's long-range vision, the program focuses on community re-entry and independence as the ideal outcome. "By providing case management that emphasizes independent problem-solving and client empowerment," says Tammy, "our goal is to improve the quality of life for our members while managing Medicaid dollars more efficiently." The program has proven remarkably effective: "We had 40 slots," Tammy continues, "and Medicaid budgeted $60,000 per patient. We're spending about $40,000. So now we can say to the state, 'Hey, do it our way. We're having good results, the clients are happier, and it saves tax dollars.'" Today there is a long waiting list for the program.

In a related effort to strengthen the continuum, 1998 also saw the establishment of CommuniCare, an improved system for patient follow-up available to patients who do not qualify for the Medicaid waiver. With the evolving technology of telemedicine, Shepherd's rehabilitation case managers could maintain regular contact with newly discharged patients, guiding their exercise programs and skills applications, and also monitoring for medical complications.

Not to be forgetful of its inpatient population, the Shepherd Building completed a $3 million facelift in 1998. Funded largely by Herbert and Lilla Gordy's generous bequest, the improved amenities included individually controlled heat and air conditioning in each room, motorized overhead patient lifts, headwalls with added patient controls, and new furniture and interior finishes. As a gesture of appreciation, Shepherd's newly renovated second floor was named the Lilla and Herbert Gordy Spinal Cord Injury Unit. A special focus of the second-floor renovation effort was the Activities of Daily Living Feature Kitchen, the specially equipped kitchen where mobility-impaired patients can improve the food-preparation skills likely to be needed after discharge. Funding for this specific part of the makeover was provided by a $27,000 gift from ING Life of Georgia/ING Southland Life Insurance Companies.

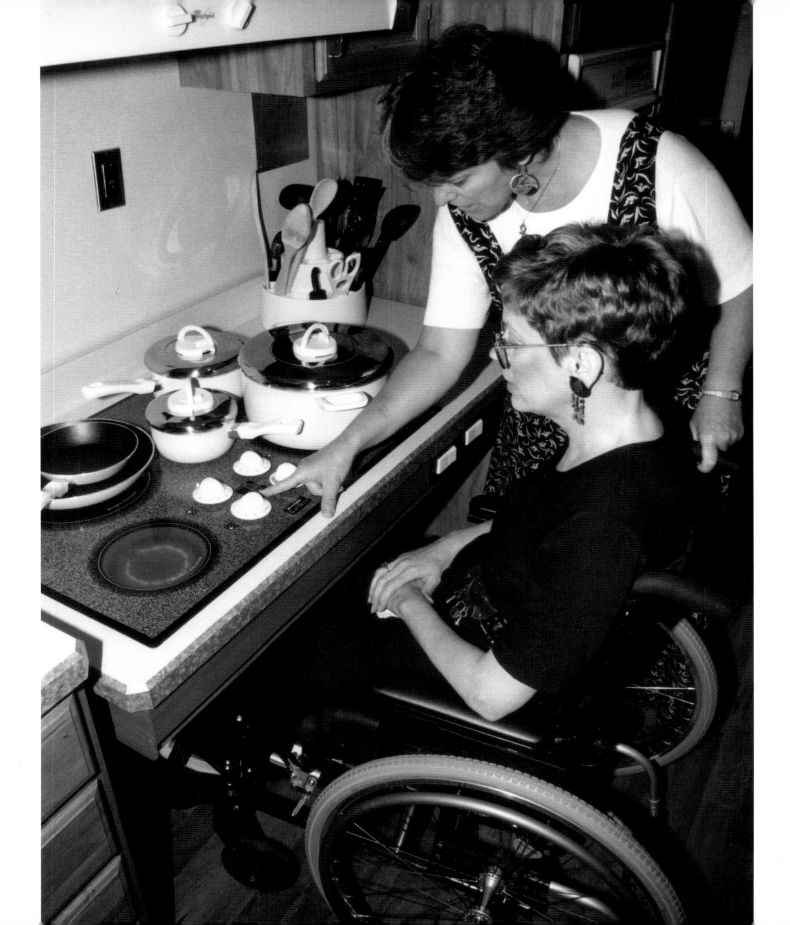

Beyond the hospital corridors, Shepherd found new ways to make its presence felt in the community in 1998. First, the center became an outspoken advocate on behalf of the Brain and Spinal Cord Injury Trust Fund, a constitutional amendment that was included on the November 3 ballot. The amendment—which did pass, much to the delight of all concerned at Shepherd—raised drunk driving fines in Georgia by 10 percent and directed that the monies be channeled into a fund for the long-term costs associated with brain and spinal cord injuries. It was estimated that the amendment would generate at least $2 million in its first year.

Second, Shepherd became the local sponsor of "On a Roll," the nation's only commercial radio talk show focusing on disability issues. Broadcast from Phoenix, Arizona, and airing in 20 cities throughout the U.S., the weekly show was picked up in Atlanta by WCNN, 680AM. In more than 200 shows, host Greg Smith has covered the kinds of topics that have always defined Shepherd's agenda—accessibility, health care, employment, and the ongoing legislative work on behalf of the disabled community.

The inspiration for the creation of Shepherd Center was not simply that James Shepherd had had to travel half way across the country to find first-class spinal cord rehabilitation; it was also that, once there, patients like James often faced the additional hardship of being out of the immediate reach and care of family and friends. The idea, originally, was to build a "local" facility for the treatment of spinal cord injury.

But 24 years later, of course, Shepherd Center was very far from being a "local" spinal cord injury hospital. In fact, by 1999, nearly half of the 800 patients admitted each year were from outside the 20-county Atlanta metropolitan area and had traveled more than two hours to get to Shepherd. Many traveled from other states; some traveled from other countries. Long aware of the housing problem faced by both day program patients living outside the Atlanta area and by the families of inpatients anxious to stay close to their loved ones, Shepherd had over the years leased a number of conveniently located apartments and also relied on the occasional "donated" apartment to help meet this urgent need.

A much better solution—and, again, typical of Shepherd's guiding spirit— was the opening in 1999 of Shepherd Place, a former office building a half-mile from the center that Shepherd purchased and renovated into a 12-unit apartment complex—fully wheelchair accessible, of course. "We made accessible housing for patients and their families a goal three years ago," said CEO Gary Ulicny. And with their generous contributions to the special Shepherd Housing Fund, he continued, "supporters who understand the value of family involvement during a

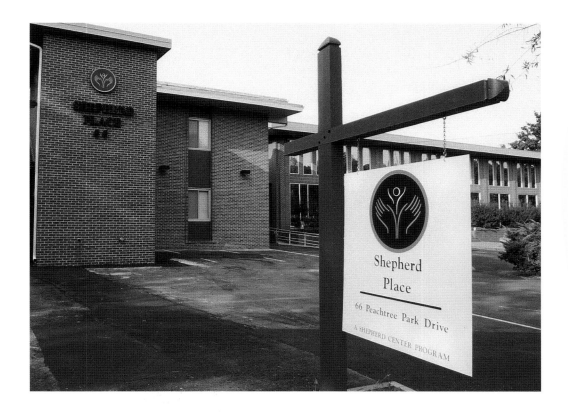

catastrophic injury have made Shepherd Place a reality."

Expressing his thanks for those early supporters and all subsequent contributors to the Housing Fund, James Shepherd said, "Family involvement and training are critical parts of recovery from a catastrophic injury of disease. We remember how important being together was to the Shepherd family in our time of crisis."

In related off-campus news, Shepherd Center received a $1.26 million HUD grant in 1999 to create Independent Communities, Inc., which would develop 14 low-income, wheelchair accessible apartments in Decatur. The new apartments, included in the multi-use redevelopment of the former Scottish Rite Children's Hospital site and adjacent property, will offer an independent living option to people with disabilities who might otherwise be forced to live in an institution after their hospital discharge. As Gary Ulicny explained, the project was entirely consistent with Shepherd's ultimate mission "to help people with disabilities regain their independence and become actively involved in community life."

Off-campus expansion in 1999 culminated with the November opening of Spring Creek House, a six-bedroom, six-bath supported living residence that goes "one step further" in Shepherd's ABI program. Also located in DeKalb County, the new facility is, in effect, an extension of Shepherd Pathways, the community-based, post-acute brain injury rehabilitation program on Clairmont Road. Another example of Shepherd's commitment to full-life rehabilitation, Spring Creek House's around-the-clock staff is there to provide assistance with such reintegration skills as money management, continuing education, and transportation.

"It's a wonderful place," says Susan Johnson, ABI program director. "Thanks to the generosity of our donors, especially the Frances Wood Wilson Foundation, we were able to purchase the house and decorate it beautifully, and we have an excellent staff there. It's a place where a brain-injured person who can't live totally independently, who just needs some help, can live indefinitely. It's really quite incredible that our support from private gifts is such that we can see things like this happen."

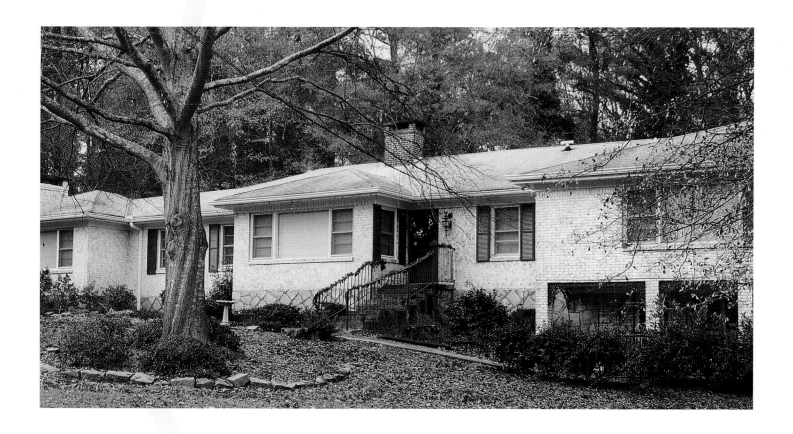

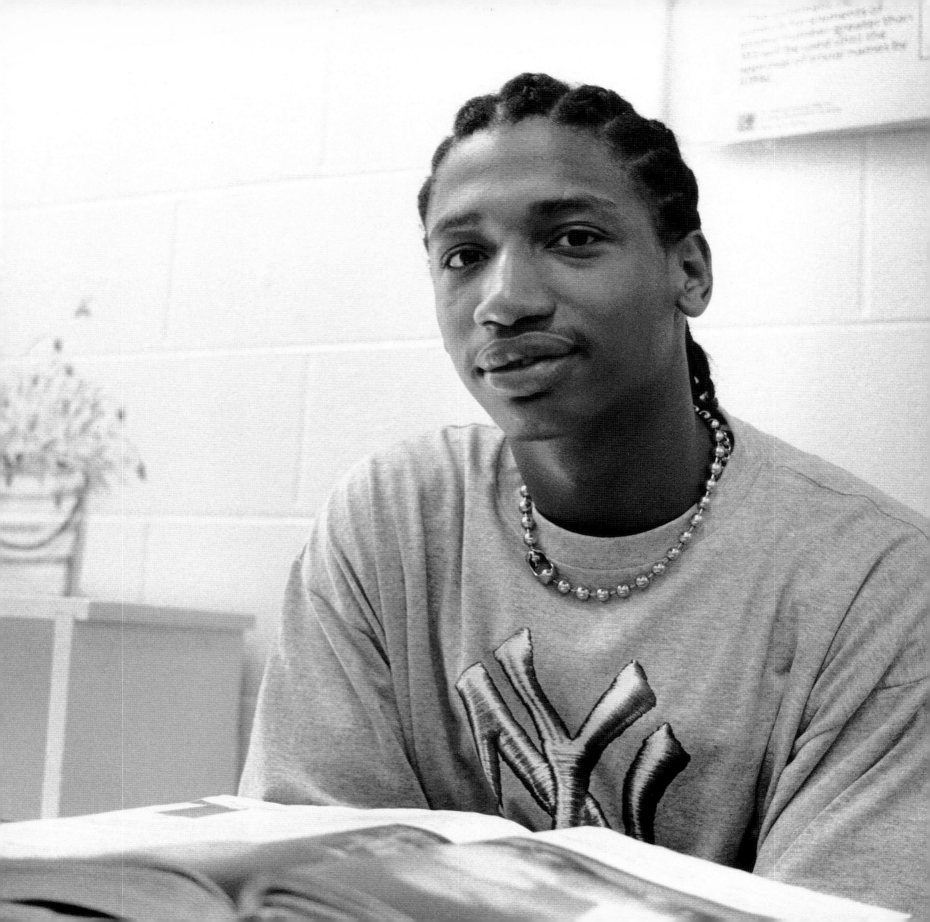

At the same time, Shepherd Center, in conjunction with Emory Healthcare, was joining a nationwide brain injury rehabilitation program called Clubhouse. On the local level, the two institutions combined to develop a not-for-profit community resource center—a Clubhouse—operated by and for people with brain injury, with minimal assistance from staff. "This is another facility providing a much-needed service," according to Dr. Leslie. "People with brain injury can have the company of others more or less in the same boat; they can be safe and enjoy themselves and at the same time be productive by exploring vocational opportunities as they further develop their cognitive and interpersonal skills."

Meanwhile, inside the hospital, Shepherd physicians and researchers continued to explore the cutting-edge rehabilitative procedures and practices that would mean optimum care for Shepherd's patients. For example, two new surgeries now available—one a "tendon transfer" procedure and the other an electrode-implant surgery—held out hope of improved hand function for patients with C-5 and C-6 spinal cord injuries. As Shepherd physiatrist Dr. Brock Bowman points out, for the right patients, the improvement can be dramatic: "A moderate amount of hand grasp and finger pinch can mean the difference between being independent in eating, cooking, shaving and other everyday tasks or in being totally dependent."

In addition, the ever-expanding array of wonders offered to patients from the assistive technology department now included Multimedia Max, a voice-activated computer that makes the wide world of the Internet—along with all the more basic computer functions—available to spinal injured patients with no hand function. "We're trying to leverage technology to get the maximum function and ability for our patients, whatever their goals are," says John Anschutz, manager of Shepherd's assistive technology center.

Before the year was out, the exceptional generosity of Shepherd's donor community was once—or twice—again in evidence. The Gordon C. Bynum, Jr. Therapeutic Recreation Endowment Fund, established in June, 1999, in memory of one of Shepherd's most devoted volunteers and friends, had received more than $150,000 before the end of the year, thanks in large measure to Shepherd's Junior Committee. And Jim Groome, tireless Shepherd volunteer since the mid-'70s and member of the board of directors since 1998, created a charitable remainder trust that designates Shepherd as a beneficiary.

As a final kudo to another remarkably productive year, Shepherd Center was named Hospital of the Year in its category for 1999. The Georgia Alliance of Community Hospitals, a state organization of not-for-profit hospitals, recognized Shepherd for improving access to health care for economically disadvantaged populations, maintaining a high level of community support, and for the quality and range of its patient services.

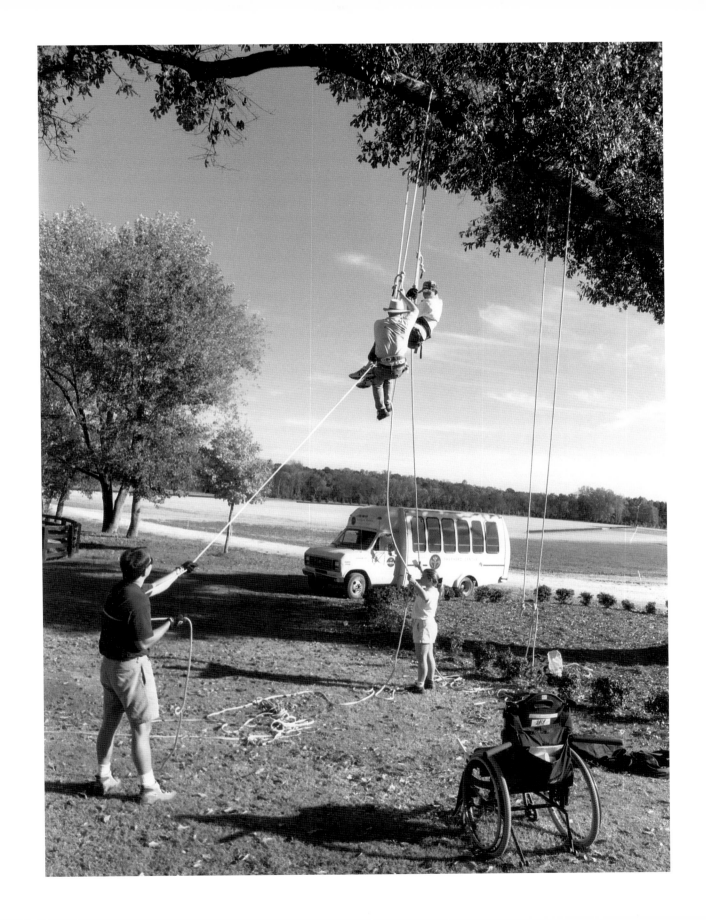

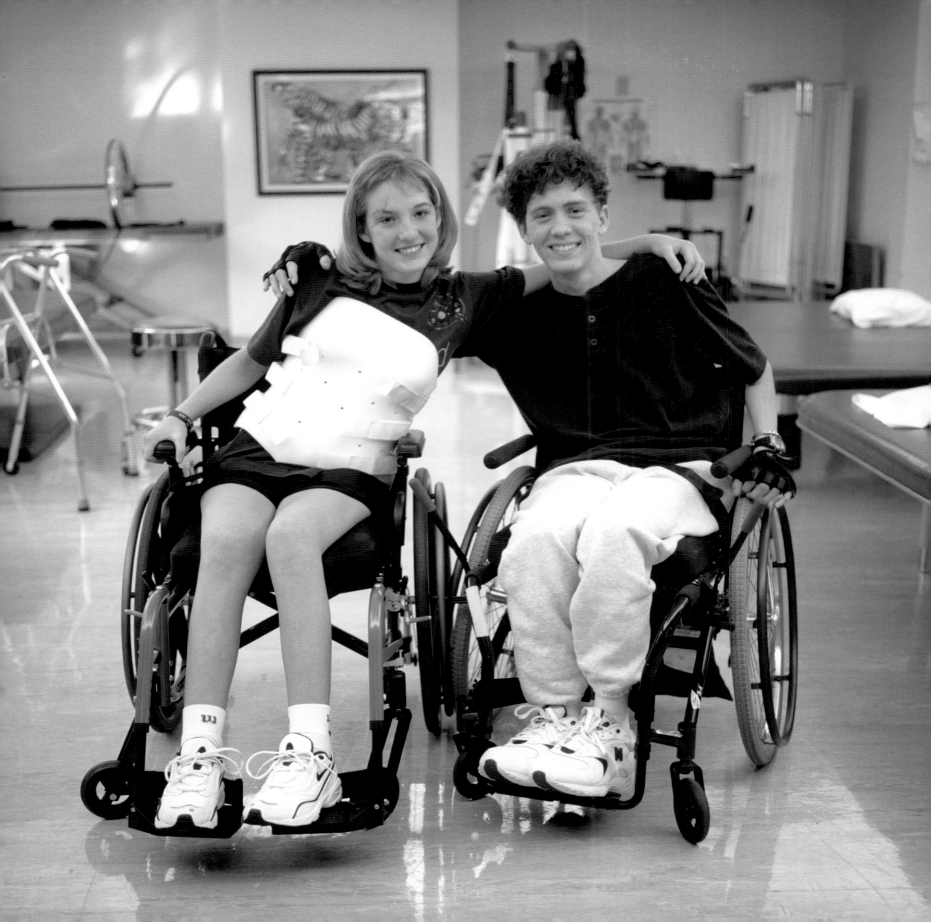

In Memorium:
Virginia Crawford
(d. August 8, 1999)

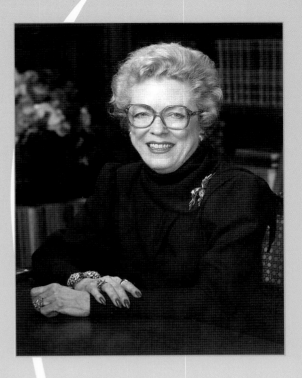

Harold Shepherd calls her, simply, "as good a friend as I ever had." If Shepherd Center had a single voice, it might just say the same thing.

Already a close friend of the Shepherd family before James Shepherd's injury, Virginia Crawford was helping build Shepherd Center before Shepherd Center existed. Alana recalls the many visits Virginia paid to James during his difficult days as a patient at Piedmont Hospital. "James was strapped on a Rotorest bed, and Virginia would lie on the floor in her nice dress holding a magazine or newspaper for him to read."

Vice president of the board of directors from the center's inception until 1995, at which time she was honored as its first honorary director, Virginia served Shepherd in every conceivable way. As a volunteer, she was a founding member of the Auxiliary, and she served on the fundraising committee for the Legendary Party every year until her death.

As a donor, her generosity knew no bounds. In 1985, her contributions made possible the creation of the Virginia Carroll Crawford Kitchen and Nutrition Centers, which constituted a revolution in hospital food service—and a fabulous amenity for Shepherd patients. In 1986, in acknowledgment of that gift as well as all of her other efforts, she was honored as Shepherd's Angel of the Year.

Virginia also served on the capital campaign committee, which successfully raised $12 million for the expansion that would become The Billi Marcus Building. Then, in 1996, yet another major gift from Virginia endowed the Virginia C. Crawford Research Institute, whose pioneering work promises to keep Shepherd on the forefront of catastrophic care for years to come.

According to James Shepherd, "As much as Virginia gave financially, she gave even more of her heart. She was a visionary who really understood what we were about, and she was instrumental in putting in place some of the most valuable pieces of our program. She had a major impact on the lives of our patients, as well as many others, through her kindness and generous spirit."

Twenty-Five Years Down, A Millennium to Go

As Shepherd Center celebrated its 25th birthday at the dawn of the new century, the big question came clearly into focus: With managed care having mandated a much less than ideal length of in-hospital stay for the catastrophically injured, how could Shepherd continue to provide its patients with the best possible rehabilitation and the greatest chance of leading productive lives as employees, homeowners, parents and community leaders? Answering the question would require, in full measure, all of the center's hallmark strengths: vision, management flexibility, technical and clinical expertise, high-powered research, and devoted community support.

Part of the answer fell into place when Shepherd Center began the year 2000 with a leap into the technological future. The center's telerehabilitation research effort received a $460,000 grant from the U.S. Department of Commerce to build an experimental Next Generation Internet (NGI) network—a computer network designed to link people with spinal cord and brain injuries to an information superhighway specific to their needs. In a wonderful example of the productive confluence of cutting-edge work in medical science, technology, and industry, Shepherd is collaborating on the project with Georgia Tech's Biomedical Interactive Technology Center, Earthlink (formerly Mindspring Enterprises), and Siemens Corporation to build the network.

The new network promises to bring into former patients' homes a wide range of high-tech services: virtual visits with Shepherd doctors and therapists via high-bandwidth videoconferencing, remote medical monitoring, and interactive multimedia instructional programs, among other marvels. According to Mike Jones, Shepherd's director of research and the lead investigator on the project, the pilot program will provide 30 recently discharged patients in the Atlanta area with two-way video and voice access to each other and to Shepherd. "The advanced technology," says Mike, "will improve Shepherd's remote medical monitoring of vital signs, medical complications, and other information important in evaluating

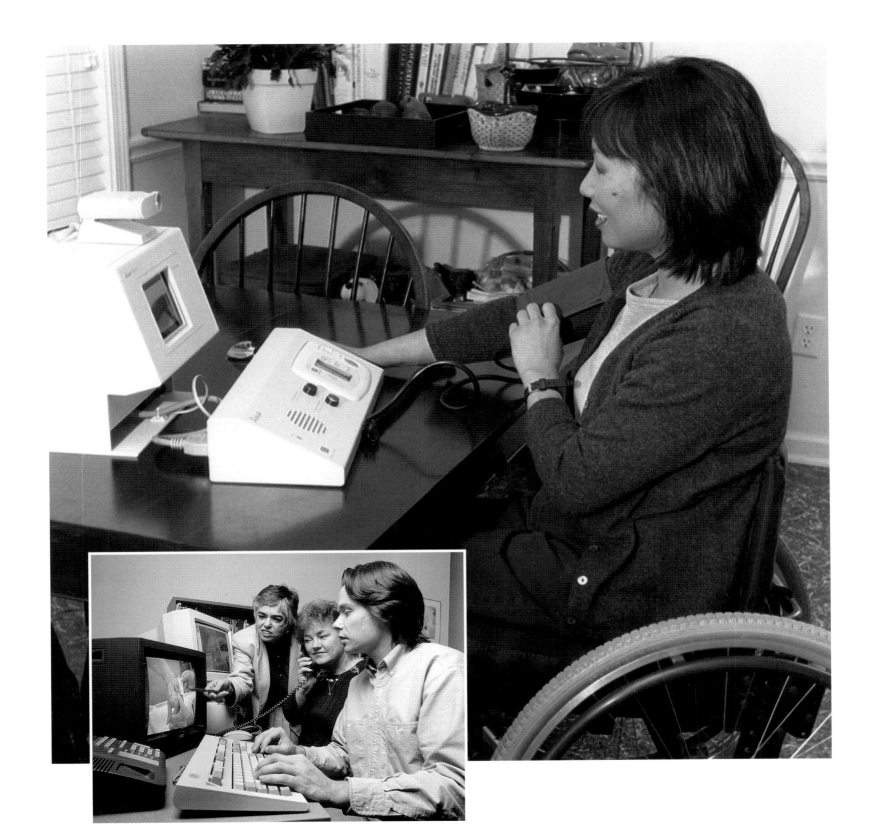

recently injured patients' recovery."

At the same time, in a wonderful instance of technological serendipity, every bed inside the hospital was being wired for Internet access thanks to a generous gift from Jamie Reynolds. Reynolds had been a patient at Shepherd after breaking his neck—an incomplete injury—in a polo accident in 1996.

Then in April came the big announcement. Billi and Bernie Marcus approved a $17.6 million grant from the Marcus Foundation—the largest single gift in Shepherd's history—to establish the Marcus Community Bridge Program, intended to provide up to 12 months of follow-up care to virtually every new patient who comes through the doors of Shepherd. Funded for eight years at $2.2 million a year, the program will offer the best possible transition-to-home services for departing patients—including telemedicine technology, vocational services, self-care education, and therapeutic recreation in clients' own communities.

The program's emphasis on home and community-based services will not only be of immediate benefit to newly discharged patients; it will help bring the insurance industry and government policy into the 21st century. According to Shepherd president and CEO Gary Ulicny, "We expect this grant to substantially improve medical outcomes and the quality of our patients' lives. Our hope is eventually to use data from this program to influence Medicaid, Medicare and private insurers to include community-based components in their health insurance plans."

The program's high-tech component—a personal computer on loan to each discharged patient, complete with access to a disability-specific Internet network and telemedicine technology—brings into clients' homes remote nurse visits via live video, assistance with equipment repair, and peer support.

"Now we'll be able to follow the patient after discharge, which of course is much sooner than it used to be," says Tammy King, who serves as director of the new program, "and we hope to be able to help people apply those skills they've learned while an inpatient very quickly. We hope to help them get back into school, back to work, back to recreation, and we want to keep them thinking right: applying those skills, avoiding skin sores and other medical complications while being productive in the community."

For Tammy, one of the center's original staffers and, most recently, the manager of ShepherdCare, the program is a tremendous step forward: "I'm totally excited," she says. "It's the perfect extension of Shepherd's whole effort. It's the natural continuation of rehabilitation, which is what I love. We never stop asking, 'How can we make it better.'"

The remarkably generous grant for the Marcus Community Bridge Program deepens Shepherd Center's already considerable gratitude to Billi and Bernie Marcus, two of the centers most loyal and devoted benefactors.

It's so rewarding when patients go off and, really, rebuild their lives, then come back and tell you, "You were a part of this."

—Tammy King
Director, Marcus Community Bridge Program

Peer Support

"As soon as my own recovery would allow," says Curtis Rodgers, who was injured in a construction accident in 1981 and underwent close to six months of rehabilitation at Shepherd, "I started volunteering to talk to new patients as they came in." For the next two years, he would be part of the loose federation of volunteers filling the increasingly important role of "peer supporters."

His motive? "I saw from my own experience how very important it is in the early stages of rehab for a patient to be able to talk to someone who has been through this, who has gone home and faced the tough issues we all face when we leave the hospital environment, where doors open automatically and a nurse is waiting at the end of a call button."

So in 1984 Curtis was among the dozen or so former patients who came together to form the officially instituted peer support program. Originally under the leadership of Judy Oviatt, peer support quickly developed into another one of those "value-added," community-supported programs that so clearly set Shepherd apart from the typical rehabilitation hospital. "It's the Shepherd philosophy," says Curtis, who became the manager of the program, "to help people reintegrate into the community as fully as possible, with the knowledge that when they leave Shepherd, it's just the beginning of the journey back. Our job is to reassure them that all the goals they had before their injury are still within their grasp if they will just reach out for them."

And like the other programs that have become so integral to Shepherd's mission, peer support has grown dramatically. "Now we have approximately 300 people in our database," says Curtis, "primarily throughout the Southeast, but also in other parts of the country." With such a wide network, virtually no one is out of reach. No matter where home is, somebody from Shepherd's program is there waiting.

Moreover, in those distant locales where a Shepherd peer supporter might not be physically present, there is now the Internet. "We set up a chat room in September 1999," says Curtis, "and now we have close to 100 on-line peer supporters, some of them even in other countries. We can post messages on any topic out there, and within a few hours somebody will reply. It's a fantastic way to reach out, to discuss and learn more, and the anonymity of the Internet can also be a plus since it avoids the possibility of embarrassment."

Today, every patient entering Shepherd's spinal cord unit is quickly made aware of the availability of peer support. Curtis explains that he normally waits until a day or two after new patients have their medical conference, then he goes in and introduces himself and the program and offers to set up a meeting with one of the peer support group. "Sometimes new patients have a difficult time seeing beyond the end of the bed," says Curtis. "They may not be in rehab right away; they may need acute medical care for a few days before they're ready for the physical requirements of our rehab program. That's a critical time to let them know that their lives will go on, that others have been through what they're going through."

From his unique perspective, the peer support program has special meaning for Curtis. "To be able to return something that was given to me 19 years ago is simply a dream come true."

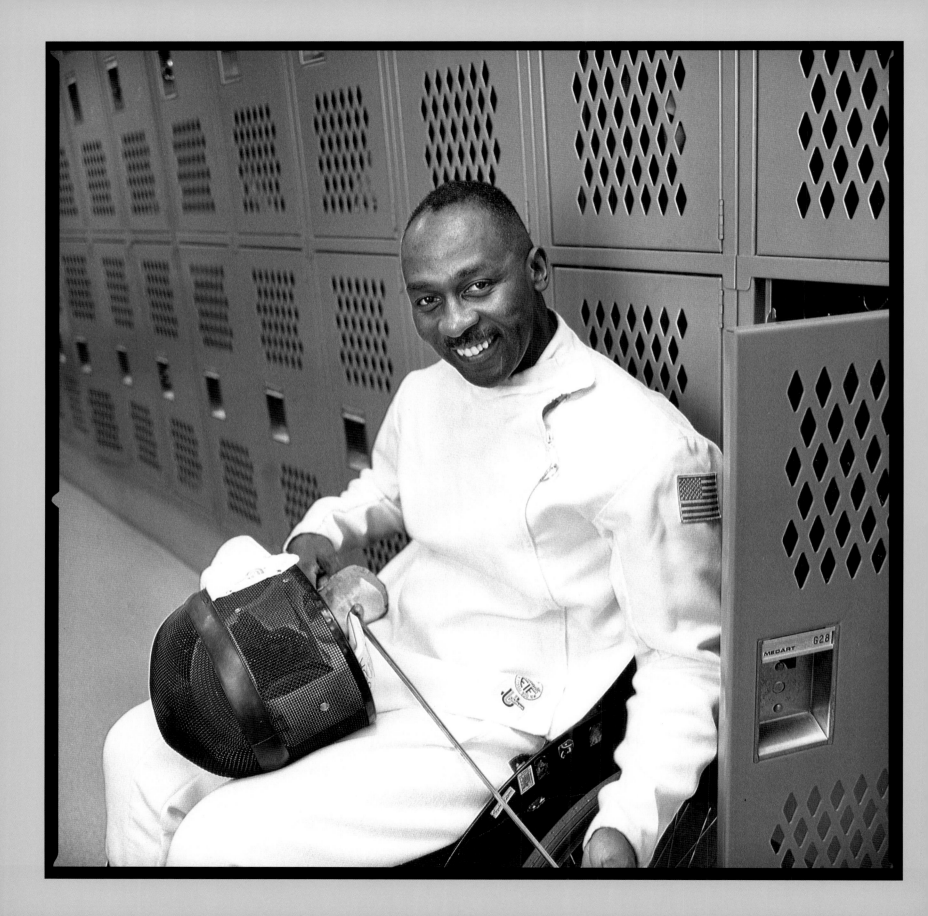

*S*ome people are born on "go."

When Curtis Lovejoy was injured in an automobile accident at the age of 29, he had already been working for Church's Fried Chicken for 15 years. In 1986, the year of the accident, he was one of the top managers in the Atlanta area, with a half dozen stores in his territory.

"I was ready to cut back on my hours and start a family with my wife, Marissa," recalls Curtis.

A car wreck on a rain-slicked highway changed those plans, but failed to diminish Curtis's spirit. He was transferred from Grady Hospital to Shepherd within hours after his accident, and Dr. Allen McDonald operated on his spine a week later. "Within a few days after the operation," says Curtis, "I was able to sit in my wheelchair and wheel myself around. I remember telling myself in the recovery room that I mustn't hold any grudges. I had to accept this injury and fight back. I had a lot to do."

Andrew Young, then mayor of Atlanta, declared December 13, 1986, Curtis Lovejoy Day. The mayor sent Curtis a proclamation and a ceremony was held at one of Curtis's stores.

"It was overwhelming," says Curtis. "My nurse, Sandy Brady, went with me, and Church's Fried Chicken even set up a Curtis Lovejoy Fund."

As it happened, though, Curtis decided to return to school rather than resume his career with Church's, and after eighteen months he completed his degree at Morris Brown College. His career goal was a job in therapeutic recreation, but his widely varied interests and inexhaustible energy have made it impossible for Curtis to do just one thing.

Take athletics, for example. "I started swimming as part of my therapy," Curtis says. "This was back before the Marcus Building was completed, and I would meet my therapist at the Y. Then, once the Marcus Building was completed, I started to practice for real."

With the amenities provided by the Marcus Building, Shepherd also started a fencing team, and Curtis discovered another passion. The result: at the 1996 Paralympic Games held in Atlanta, Curtis was selected as an alternate on both the U.S. swimming and fencing teams. But Curtis's athletic career was just getting started. At the 2000 Games in Sydney, Curtis not only competed in swimming and fencing events, he returned to Atlanta with two gold medals in swimming.

But make no mistake: the considerable time required for these endeavors does not impinge upon Curtis's full slate of community service. He works with both the Boy Scouts and Cub Scouts, he is a deacon in his church, and he is a sought-after motivational speaker for youth groups, churches, and corporations. He particularly enjoys his work with BUCKS, a church-sponsored, community-targeted men's organization that focuses on self-esteem issues. He has served on the Mayor's Disability Council, the Multicultural and Atlanta Task Forces. Such tireless work has brought him well-deserved recognition, including the coveted WXIA-TV Channel 11 Community Service Award.

And there is still the work he does at Shepherd, where he coaches the swim team and has for many years been one of the center's most loyal and devoted peer supporters.

"It's the most humanitarian thing we can do," says Curtis about working as a peer supporter. "We need to show more love to one another and to spread that love to those in need."

(Thanks to Jennifer Grizzle's profile of Curtis, "On the Move!" in Spinal Column, Fall 1994, pp. 4-5.)

Curtis

Lovejoy

"I tell patients that the sky's the limit, and that they all have the same opportunities I have."

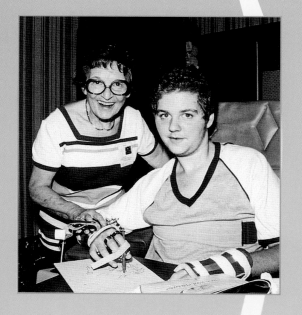

In Memorium:
Martha (Marty) Church
(d. December 27, 1999)

Marty Church, dearly remembered as the driving force behind "Pecans on Peachtree," began a second career of volunteering when she retired from teaching in 1972. By 1983, when she was recognized by United Way as the Metropolitan Atlanta Volunteer of the Year, she had put in more than 4,000 volunteer hours at Shepherd, in every imaginable capacity.

In 1985, Marty was one of eleven honorees of the WXIA-TV 11-Alive community service program "The Ones Who Care." Characteristically, she requested that her $1,000 award be given to Shepherd in order to launch the Patient Equipment Fund..

In 1986, Marty, Alana Shephered, and Katharine Jones became the first recipients of the Auxiliary's Award for Excellence, established in honor of founding board member Alana.

At its spring luncheon in 1989, the Auxiliary recognized Marty for her longtime service by naming in her honor the Martha Jane Church Conference Room, funded by a portion of the Auxiliary's annual gift to Shepherd, located on the first floor of the Shepherd Building. Still working hard on behalf of Shepherd Center seven years later, Marty was honored as Shepherd's Angel of the Year in 1996.

She was a formidable saleswoman even from her mobile scooter," noted Alana Shepherd. "And she never slowed down. She was always talking, selling, and enlisting new volunteers." Marty still holds the record for the most volunteer hours given to Shepherd — 5,647—a record not likely to be broken.

And finally, still addressing the question of the long-term needs of patients post-discharge, Shepherd this year initiated the ExtendedCare program. According to its innovative provisions, patients receive in-hospital rehabilitation, outpatient day program rehabilitation, durable medical equipment, outpatient visits, home health and attendant care, medications and supplies, telemedicine services and other services deemed necessary by the treatment team—all at one all-inclusive rate, making it attractive to insurance providers.

According to Mitch Fillhaber, vice president of marketing and managed care, "The progress patients make in rehabilitation can be lost without the critically important post-discharge phase, which reinforces skills learned in the hospital and applies them to a person's daily life. Studies show that the more thorough post-discharge rehabilitation people receive, the more independent they become and the lower the long-term cost to insurers."

A mark of Shepherd's creative problem solving, ExtendedCare represents the first time a rehabilitation provider has combined inpatient and outpatient services and offered them for a fixed price.

In addition to the 25th anniversary of Shepherd Center, the year 2000 also marked the 10th anniversary of the Americans with Disabilities Act (ADA) and the 25th anniversary of the Individuals with Disabilities Education Act (IDEA), two pieces of landmark legislation on behalf of people with disabilities. As summertime approached, thanks to the efforts of Initiative 2000, a group of organizers who had been at work for three years, more than 500 cities around the country were planning events that would "Renew the Pledge" of ADA and unify in a two-months-long celebration the nationwide community of people with disabilities.

The highlight of the celebration was the 24-city, Spirit of ADA Torch Relay, from June 11 through August 7, starting in Houston and concluding at the United Nations in New York City. For Shepherd Center, one of the national sponsors of the relay, the big day came on July 20, when a crowd of 300 supporters gathered in the center's parking lot for the start of the relay's seven-mile trek through downtown Atlanta.

Shepherd's advocacy coordinator Mark Johnson, one of the original members of Initiative 2000 and a chief architect of the relay, kicked off the event by telling the assembled crowd, "None of this happens unless everyone recognizes everyone else's value. Everybody counts. This has all been about acceptance, so we have to work on acceptance."

Meanwhile, Alana Shepherd carried the torch through the throng of patients, staff, and members of the disabled community, many of whom had tears in their eyes as they reached out to touch it. "Just look at their faces," she said. "It's so neat. It's not just the law. People are looking beyond the law to what's the right thing to do."

"We're here to celebrate our civil rights," added James Shepherd, "and to use this event as an opportunity to celebrate the achievements of people with disabilities."

During its Atlanta leg, the torch relay made a number of stops: the First Presbyterian Church, one of the first in the city to become accessible to the disabled, the Carter Center, the Martin Luther King Jr. Center, and, finally, the State Capitol, where Governor Roy Barnes declared July the "Spirit of ADA Month in Georgia."

One month later another very special 25th anniversary celebration was held at Shepherd. In the corridor near the main elevator lobby on the first floor of the

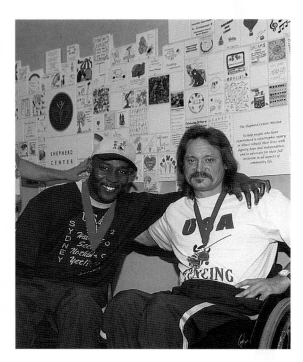

L-R: Curtis Lovejoy and Roy Day, Jr.

Shepherd Building, the "Tile Wall" was unveiled. Entitled "A View of Shepherd," the tile wall—16 feet long and four feet high—consists of approximately 250 ceramic tiles decorated with original art by Shepherd employees and volunteers. Hosted by founding board members James Shepherd and Alana Shepherd, medical director Dr. David Apple, and president and CEO Gary Ulicny, the event was inspired by a quarter-century of staff dedication to Shepherd Center's mission to provide excellence in catastrophic care. The tiles will remain as a remembrance of the anniversary as well as a permanent expression of thanks to those whose work has made the center such a remarkable success.

Gary Ulicny opened the ceremony by remarking that "Shepherd has an energy and a vibrancy that you just don't find at other places, and that is truly due to our employees. So the wall is an opportunity for our employees to have a lasting legacy. We're glad you're here and we're proud of all you've done over the past 25 years. We're proud of each and every one of you."

Added James Shepherd: "The real honor is to look around and see the faces of people who have been with us for the whole 25 years—too many to name here. And it's not so much that I'd like to say thank you for what you've done for the center, but more for what you've done for the patients that have come through these doors. We've seen about 20,000 people come through here, and you've helped restore hope into their lives; you've helped them go back out and get jobs, have families . . . and I just want to say we are all grateful for what you all have done."

Alana Shepherd agreed that it was a joy to see the long-time employees, but noted, "When you started is not as important as what you are doing now. Any of you could work anyplace in the city, but you choose to work here with these patients."

And finally, in the words of Dr. Apple, "This wall represents the countless hours of caring, compassion and clinical excellence our staff has demonstrated over the last 25 years. Shepherd Center is deeply indebted to the hundreds of employees, volunteers, and medical staff whose remarkable dedication has restored the dignity, hope and lives of thousands of patients. Thank you."

Among the guests singled out for their contributions to the center were Roy Day, Jr., an original board member, and Curtis Lovejoy, former patient, volunteer and peer supporter—both of whom would soon be representing Shepherd, and the U.S., in the Paralympic Games in Sydney, Australia. Roy, originally injured in 1972 and in recent years the captain of Shepherd's fencing team, offered his own assessment of the 25-year achievement: "When people ask me how Shepherd happened, I tell them Alana built it brick by brick."

In fact, Roy and Curtis were but two of six Shepherd athletes who qualified for the 2000 Paralympics, prompting therapeutic recreation department manager Mike Hufstetler to remark, "I don't know of any other facility in the country

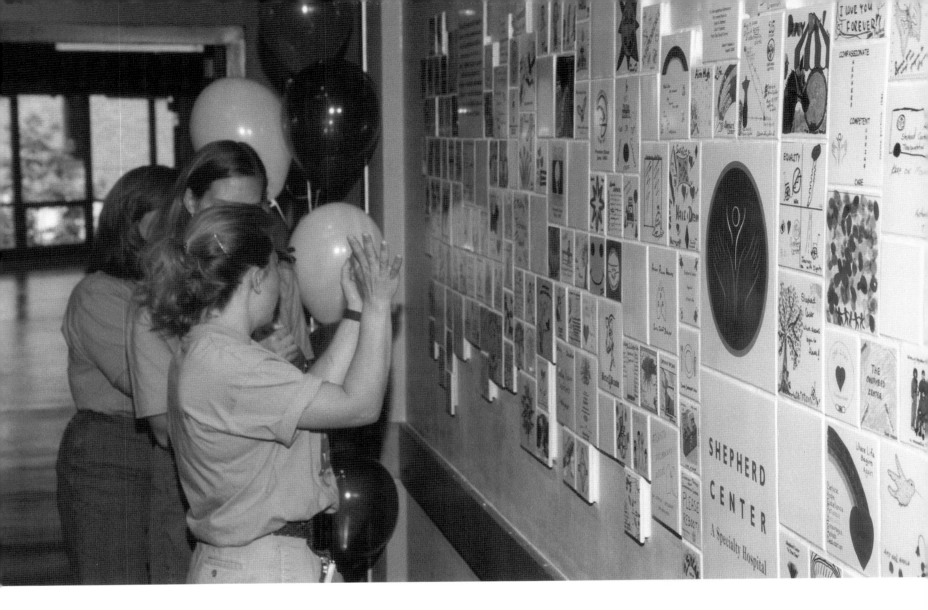

that has this many athletes on the U.S. team." In addition to Curtis (who qualified in both fencing and swimming), the other members of Roy's fencing team included Scott Rodgers, Carol Hickey and Lisa Lanier. Bert Burns, a gold medallist in the '92 Games in Barcelona, qualified for the U.S. track team.

Roy proved prophetic. Uncertain what the prospects for the fencing team might be, he nonetheless guaranteed that Curtis would medal in swimming: "After all, he set two world records during qualifying." Sure enough, Curtis brought home gold medals in both the 100-meter freestyle and the 50-meter freestyle. And though Shepherd's other Paralympians did not medal, the significance of the experience was not diminished. "The great thing is to be able to represent Shepherd Center and our country in such a tremendous event," said Roy.

139

In September 2000 came another milestone event – the opening of Shepherd Pain Center, offering pain management and rehabilitation for people experiencing acute and chronic pain from spinal injuries and neuromuscular disorders, post polio syndrome, degenerative disc disease, complex regional pain syndrome (RSD), fibromyalgia, cancer, and back surgery.

Located in 4,600 square feet of medical office space across Peachtree Road from Shepherd Center, the new pain treatment center offers a multidisciplinary approach, treating pain with a variety of methods – from biofeedback therapy and nerve blocks to surgically implanted devices and psychological care.

Another activity that began as the year came to a close was the search for a new full-time medical director for the MS Center at Shepherd. Dr. Ben Wade Thrower, an advocate of early MS treatments, accepted the position and planned to begin seeing Shepherd patients. Dr. Thrower comes from the Holy Family Hospital MS Center in Spokane, Washington, where he has served as the medical director since 1999.

Dr. Thrower received his medical degree from the University of Florida College of Medicine in 1988. Upon completing an internship in internal medicine, he worked on his residency in neurology at the University of Texas Health Sciences Center at San Antonio. Board-certified in neurology with a special interest in multiple sclerosis and clinical research, Dr. Thrower has been in practice for over ten years, and concentrating on MS patients exclusively for the past two years.

One of the anniversary year's great highlights occurred on October 14 when Field Day, an original and cherished Shepherd tradition, was revived after a 12-year hiatus. On one of those perfect autumn days, the sun shone in a deep blue sky, the maple trees around the parking lot of the Marcus Building glowed bright orange, and the grounds were festooned with helium-filled balloons in Shepherd's trademark blue, gold, and white colors. A DJ spun rock music into the celebration-charged atmosphere.

The morning was given to outdoor events: the basketball toss, the obstacle course (which was negotiated by former patient Robert Antonisse in the winning time of 32.59 seconds), and the ever-popular Dunk-'em Machine. Dr. David Apple, Dr. Donald Leslie, VP of Development Dell Sikes, CFO Steve Holleman, and VP for Operations Jason Shelnutt all took their turns getting dropped into the cold tank, but the line of dunkers lengthened noticeably when president and CEO Gary Ulicny took his seat over the watery abyss. Fearlessly taunting the contestants with jibes like "Rubber arm!" and "Is that your best shot?" Gary took the plunge time after time – in several instances at the hands of his own children.

After a lunch catered by Chick-fil-A, the action moved into the Livingston

Gymnasium, which was jam-packed for the much-anticipated "Doctors' Relay." The first of several heats featured Dr. Brock Bowman's team against the team anchored by Dr. Dave Apple, who wore not only the required blindfold but an Indian chief's headdress as well. As board member Sara Chapman commented on the sideline, "The most fun anybody has here is dressing Dr. Apple up and making him look ridiculous."

The success of the day was measured not only by the great time had by the patients and staff in attendance, but especially by the almost 100 former patients who returned to Shepherd for the event. The soul of this group was typified by Tim Evatt, a 1986 graduate who remembered well the Field Days of years past and was on hand again in the year 2000. A college student when he was injured falling out of a tree, Tim returned to school at Clemson University, then went on to law school, and today works as an attorney for social services in Anderson, South Carolina. "My great mentor when I was at Shepherd," says Tim, "was [founding board member] Dave Webb. I have an autographed picture of him hanging in my office. He gave me so much encouragement and so many words of wisdom, and I try to pass them along whenever I can to others who find themselves in this situation."

That Tim, 14 years after his days as a patient here, would make the three-hour trip from Anderson to Atlanta to be part of this special day speaks volumes about the spirit that has guided Shepherd Center for a quarter of a century.

The year – and the quarter-century – came to a fitting close with the announcement that Shepherd had been recognized as one of the country's top rehabilitation hospitals, according to a survey by *U.S. News & World Report* in its annual edition of "America's Best Hospitals."

This gratifying tribute at the conclusion of Shepherd Center's milestone 25th anniversary year underscores the very special nature of the place and the people who have built it. What a journey! That the unlikely dream of a small handful of people could have become a reality far beyond the imagining of those original dreamers seems simply miraculous.

Today, Shepherd Center's mission is "to help people who have experienced a catastrophic injury or disease, which has resulted in a temporary or permanent disability, rebuild their lives with dignity, hope and independence, advocating for their full inclusion in all aspects of community life." The thousands of patients who have been embraced by that mission are a reminder of the great deeds that can be accomplished in the service of good.

As the new millennium opens, let this celebratory volume close with the words of the three people most closely identified with Shepherd Center and all that it stands for.

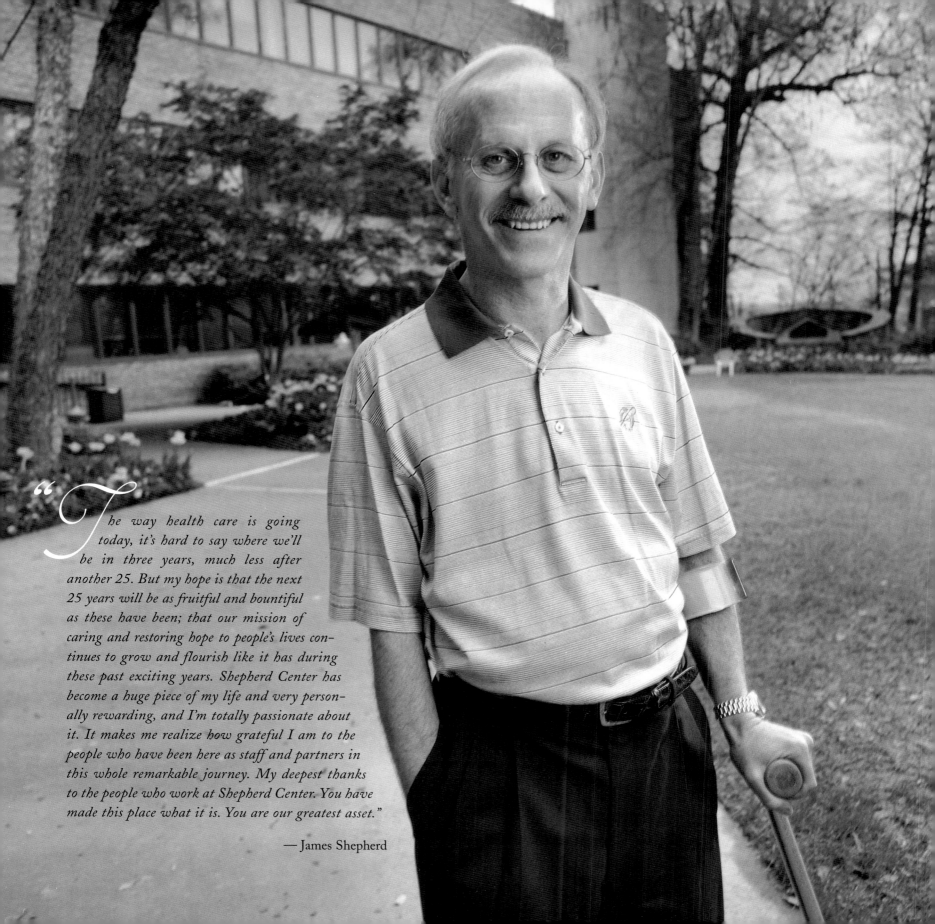

"*The way health care is going today, it's hard to say where we'll be in three years, much less after another 25. But my hope is that the next 25 years will be as fruitful and bountiful as these have been; that our mission of caring and restoring hope to people's lives continues to grow and flourish like it has during these past exciting years. Shepherd Center has become a huge piece of my life and very personally rewarding, and I'm totally passionate about it. It makes me realize how grateful I am to the people who have been here as staff and partners in this whole remarkable journey. My deepest thanks to the people who work at Shepherd Center. You have made this place what it is. You are our greatest asset.*"

— James Shepherd

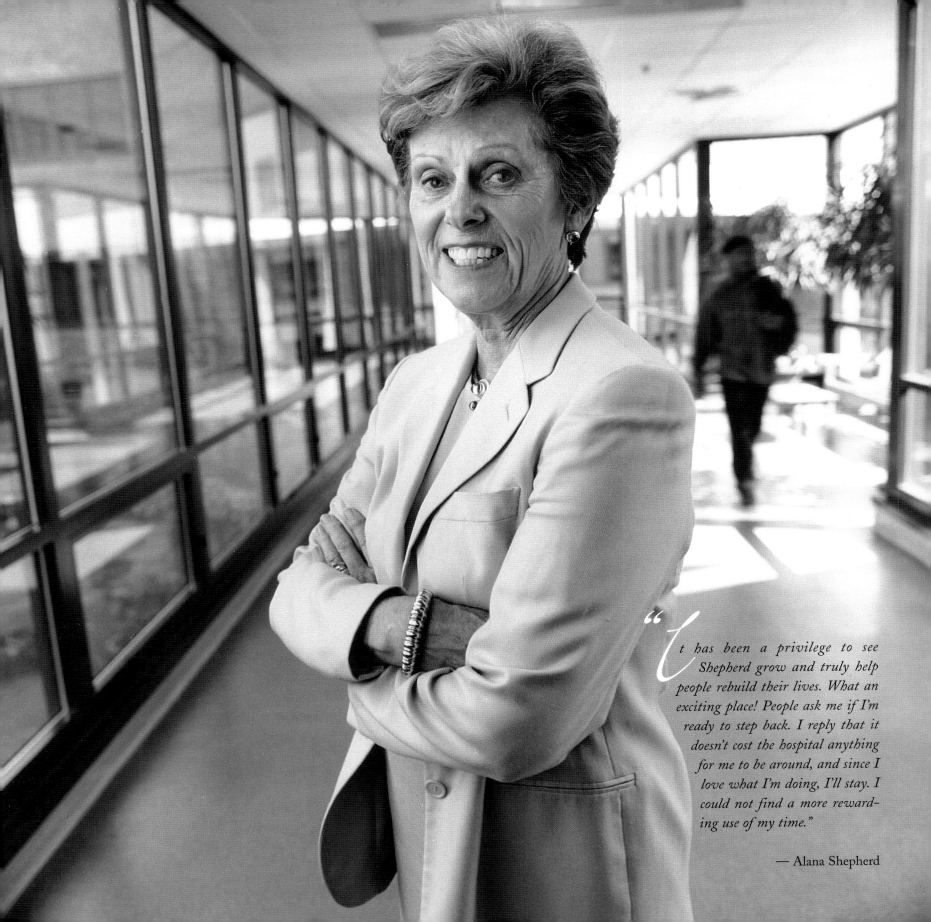

"It has been a privilege to see Shepherd grow and truly help people rebuild their lives. What an exciting place! People ask me if I'm ready to step back. I reply that it doesn't cost the hospital anything for me to be around, and since I love what I'm doing, I'll stay. I could not find a more rewarding use of my time."

— Alana Shepherd

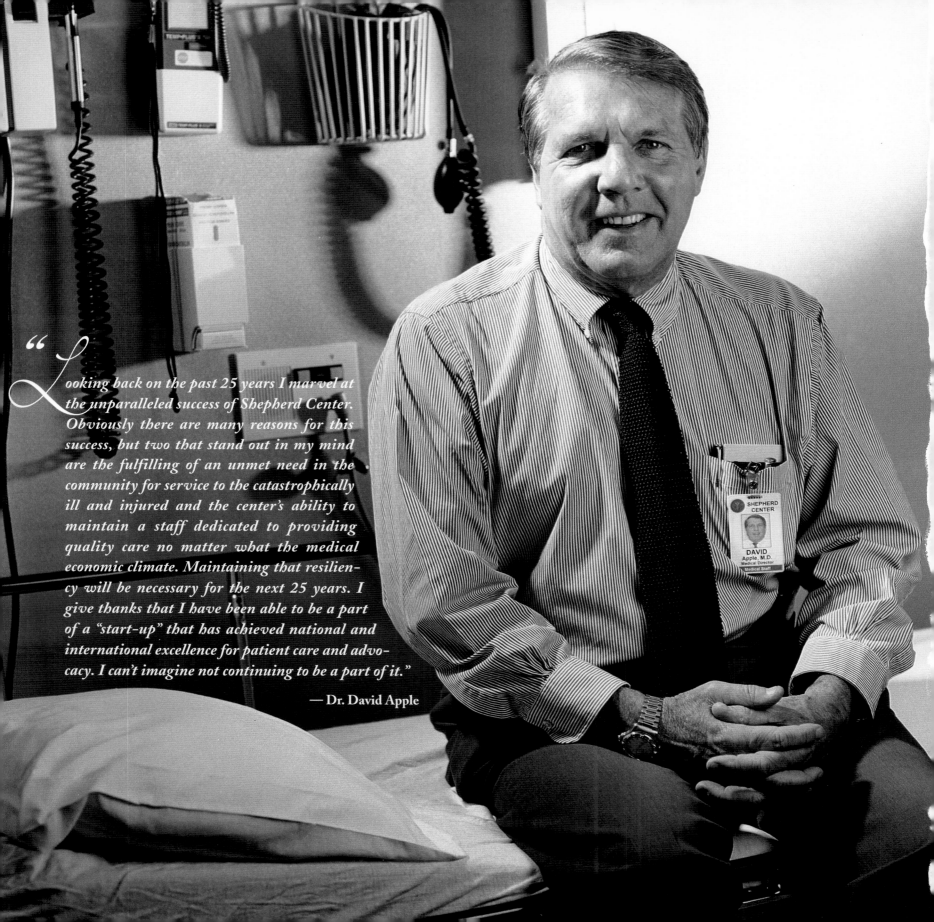

"*Looking back on the past 25 years I marvel at the unparalleled success of Shepherd Center. Obviously there are many reasons for this success, but two that stand out in my mind are the fulfilling of an unmet need in the community for service to the catastrophically ill and injured and the center's ability to maintain a staff dedicated to providing quality care no matter what the medical economic climate. Maintaining that resiliency will be necessary for the next 25 years. I give thanks that I have been able to be a part of a "start-up" that has achieved national and international excellence for patient care and advocacy. I can't imagine not continuing to be a part of it.*"

— Dr. David Apple

Epilogue: Into the Future

Since its founding in 1975, Shepherd Center has grown in size and distinction, from a six-bed unit serving people with spinal cord injuries to an innovator in acute catastrophic care, rehabilitation and research, the premiere spinal cord injury facility in the country, the largest brain injury rehabilitation program in the state of Georgia, the largest Multiple Sclerosis (MS) Center in the nation, and the catalyst for the Shepherd/Harvard MS Research collaboration.

But such growth and success has incurred inevitable costs. The facilities are suffering under the weight of increased use, with overcrowded areas for patients, staff and volunteers, and inadequate parking. Vital programs that significantly impact each patient's successful recovery are seriously threatened by the pressures of the managed care environment. Now more than ever, with much shorter inpatient stays, there is a need to follow patients after discharge when they return home. And research and education programs are poised to make great strides, but will not move forward without significant resources to secure their future.

Faced with these challenges, Shepherd Center's board of directors unanimously agreed to address the most urgent needs of the Center through a $60 million capital and endowment campaign. Led by Honorary Chairman Bernie Marcus (founder of The Home Depot and member of Shepherd's board of directors), along with Co-Chairs Arthur M. Blank (founder of The Home Depot), Alana Shepherd (founding member of Shepherd's board of directors), and David M. Ratcliffe (President and CEO of Georgia Power Company), this strategic campaign will strive to meet three over-riding goals:

- Help to ensure Shepherd Center's successful future by increasing its modest endowment from $8 million to $38 million over a five-year period.
- Allow the Center to expand its services, including new medical services, research, and much needed follow-up support to patients as they return to the community.
- Respond to pressures on physical space by revitalizing the Shepherd Center campus.

Marking the Center's 25th anniversary, this capital and endowment campaign will provide a solid foundation for the work of the next quarter-century and allow Shepherd Center to reach new heights in patient care, research and advocacy for people with disabilities.

Index

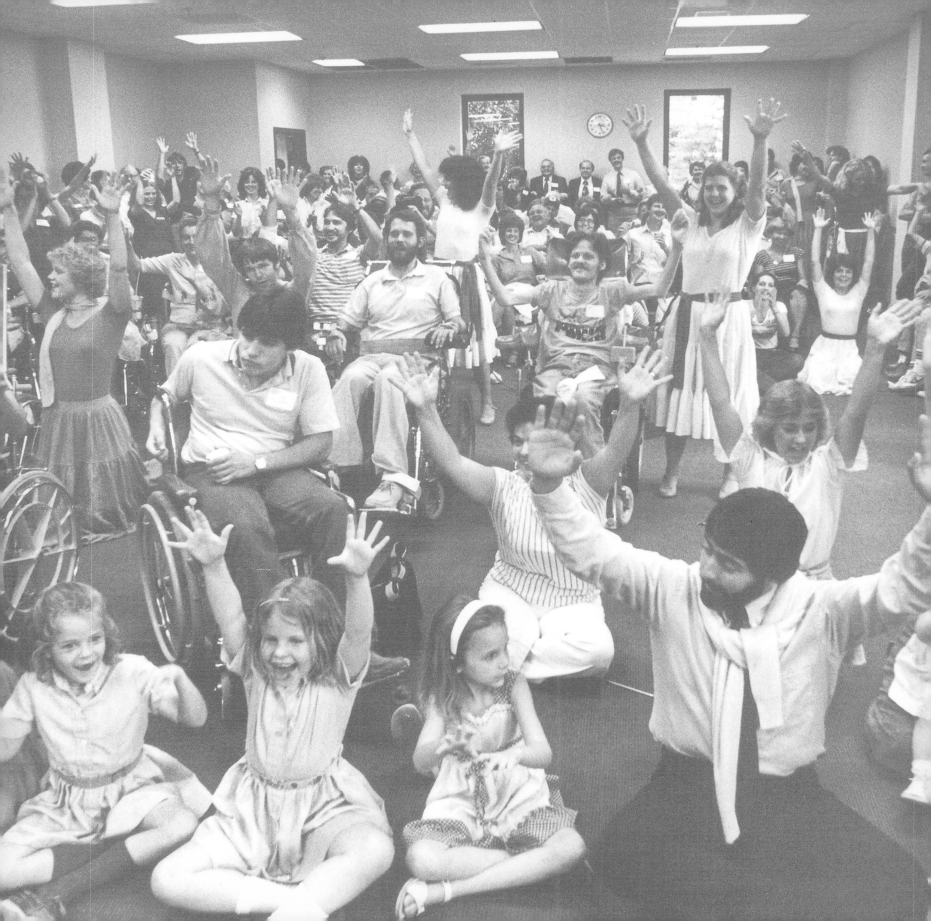

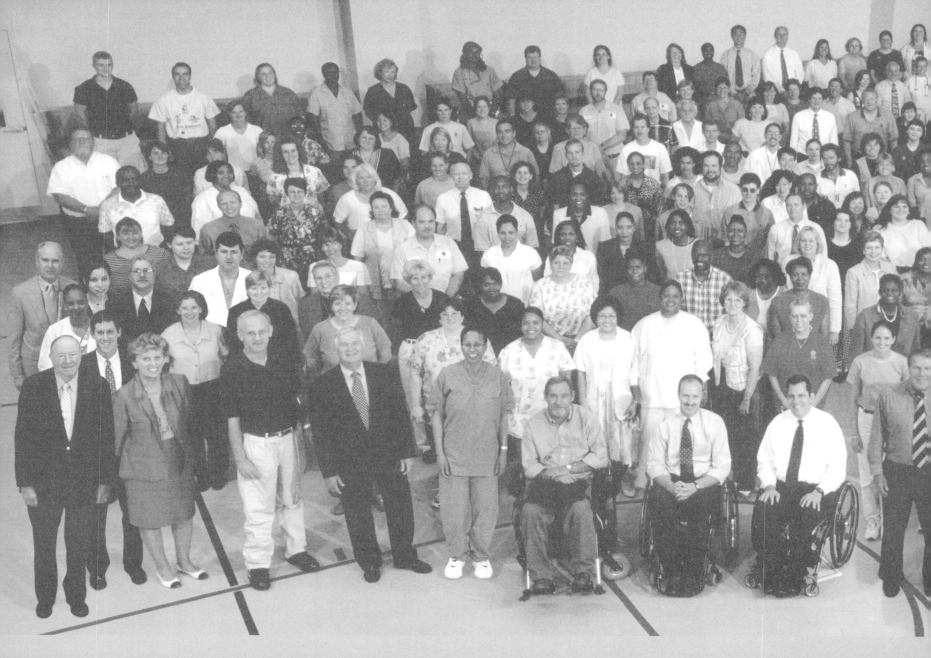